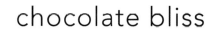

chocolate bliss

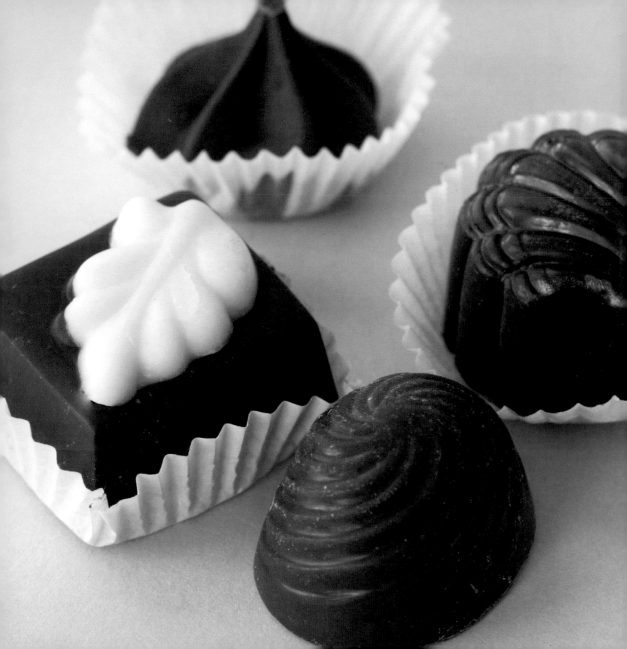

chocolate bliss

sensuous recipes, spa treatments,
and other divine indulgences

susie norris

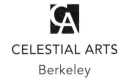

CELESTIAL ARTS

Berkeley

Copyright © 2009 by Susie Norris
Photographs copyright © 2009 by Jennifer Martiné

Published in the United States by Celestial Arts, an imprint of the Crown Publishing Group, a division of Random House, Inc., New York.
www.crownpublishing.com
www.tenspeed.com

Celestial Arts and the Celestial Arts colophon are registered trademarks of Random House, Inc.

Page v: Chocolates courtesy of Mona Lisa Food Products, Hendersonville, NC.
Pages 72–73: Chocolates courtesy of PCB Création, Benfeld, France.
Page 98: Artisan gift box courtesy of Nashville Wraps, Nashville, TN.
Page 131: *Peonies and Chocolate Pot* reproduced with permission of Carol Tarzier, www.tarzier.com.

Library of Congress Cataloging-in-Publication Data

Norris, Susie.
 Chocolate bliss : sensuous recipes, spa treatments, and other divine indulgences / by Susie Norris.
 p. cm.
 Includes bibliographical references and index.
 Summary: "A celebration of all things chocolate: every type and flavor, its health and beauty benefits, origins and ecological influences, and tasting, gifting, and baking"—Provided by publisher.
 1. Cookery (Chocolate) 2. Chocolate. I. Title.

TX767.C5N666 2009
641.3'374—dc22

2009015592

ISBN 978-1-58761-347-0

Printed in China

Design by Betsy Stromberg

10 9 8 7 6 5 4 3 2 1

First Edition

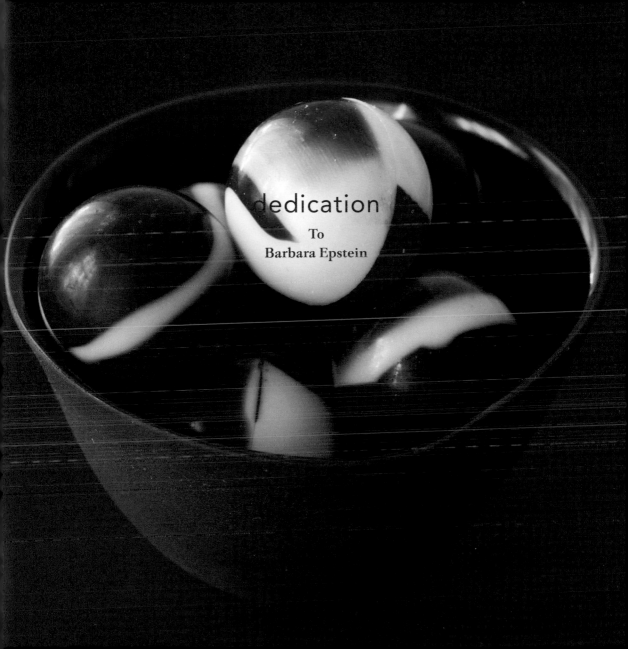

dedication

To
Barbara Epstein

contents

3 good works 73

HOW YOU CAN HELP CHOCOLATE

The Trees ✧ The People ✧ Giving Back to Chocolate ✧
Earthy Recipes: From Chili to Cheesecake

4 share the love 99

THE GIFT OF CHOCOLATE

The Chocolate-Covered Holidays ✧ Birthdays: How to Make a Great
Birthday Cake ✧ Gifting Recipes: From Cupcakes to White Chocolate Roses

acknowledgments

I am grateful to these fine chocolate professionals, authors, and chefs who gave me access, information, and inspiration: Carole Bloom, Kristy Choo of Jin Patisserie, Joshua Needleman of Chocolate Springs Cafe, Ken Givich and Gary Guittard of Guittard Chocolate Company, Elaine Gonzalez, Clay Gordon of The Chocolate Life, Stephan Iten of Felchlin Chocolate, Andre Krump of TasteTV, Maribel Leiberman of Marie Belle, Tony Lydgate of Steelgrass Farm, Ray Major of Artisan Confections, Katrina Markoff of Vosges-Haut Chocolat, Derek Pho, Eric Martinet, and Laurent Pages of Barry Callebaut, Alice Medrich, Alexander Morozoff of *Cocoaroma* magazine, Nathan Sato of Malie Kai Chocolates, Michael Schneider of *Dessert Professional* magazine, the late Robert Steinberg of Scharffen Berger Chocolate Maker, Michael Recchiuti of Recchiuti Confections, Marilyn Tausend of Culinary Adventures, Inc., and Jacques Torres of Chocolate Haven. My thanks to all of you and to the hundreds of artisan chocolatiers who keep our business so dynamic. Thanks also to the students, chef/instructors, and staff of California School of Culinary Arts, particularly Chef Joshua Orlando and Chef Norma Salazar.

I am also grateful to my agent, Betsy Amster, for her insightful work and wisdom on this project. Ten Speed Press and Celestial Arts provided many guiding lights:

extraordinary editor Lisa Westmoreland, acquirer Lorena Jones, designer Betsy Stromberg, photographer Jennifer Martiné, food stylist Julie Smith, and props stylist Theresa McNulty. Thank you all for your professionalism and creativity.

Friends and family provided the joie de vivre necessary for this job. My father-in-law Jason Epstein (author, editor, and entrepreneur) brought the exuberant cookbook author Maida Heatter to my house for dinner, and she brought along a box of Palm Beach Brownies. This trio (editor, author, brownie) inspired my professional pursuit of the pastry arts, for which I am indeed grateful. Contributions from my three children—Sam, Natalie, and Thomas—as well as those by my dessert-tasting and chocolate-loving friends, are everywhere. Thanks to my mom and dad for passing along the journalistic spirit, and to the sister/writers in my family, Frances Norris and Helen Epstein, for their knowing encouragement. Deepest thanks to my husband, Jacob Epstein, for the years he has served as my writing coach and finest friend.

Chocolate—elixir made from the fruit of the cacao tree (pronounced ka-KOW) known by its scientific name *Theobroma cacao* or "food of the gods."

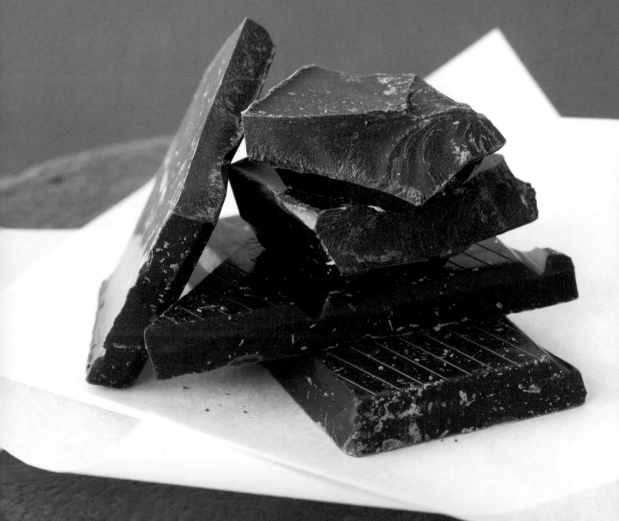

introduction

I am a pastry chef, chocolatier, culinary school teacher, and Snickers Bar sneaker. My never-ending adoration of chocolate leads me to many cultures and to many fellow enthusiasts. I offer this book in celebration of all the ways chocolate—part health food, part soul food—brings us bliss.

Chocolate is more than a fruit, more than a candy, more than a drink, more than a sweet dessert. It is the third largest commodity on the global exchange after sugar and coffee, commanding over $40 billion in annual trading revenues. Fifty million people worldwide work hard to bring cacao plants to fruition and the fruit to our hands. Chocolate generates an estimated $80 billion per year for international companies such as Cargill, Nestlé, Hershey's, Cadbury, and Mars. Its production has sustained the economies of Indonesia, Brazil, Venezuela, and numerous African nations. In addition to its commercial strength, chocolate's history is full of drama. It nourished Mayan warriors, enriched Aztec kings, infuriated Spanish priests, enslaved the downtrodden, puzzled doctors, scandalized ladies, delighted soldiers, charmed children, and spawned huge corporate empires. Its power is miraculous; it is truly the food of the gods.

The recipes in this book celebrate chocolate's flavors, history, and global appeal. They include traditional desserts, cakes, and candies, a few savory dishes, and some ideal approaches for the health-conscious chocolate lover. We'll explore chocolate's potential in the fight against deforestation and global warming and the many traditions for giving chocolate as a gift. We'll see why giving the dark food of the gods brings such brightness to the world.

a word about techniques and tools

If you can make a batch of chocolate chip cookies, you can make any recipe in this book. Baking and working with chocolate are not hard, just specific. Like most pastry chefs, my background comes from the French *pâtisserie* tradition, which involves formal procedures, formulas, and many French terms. The recipes here are designed to bring some classic French techniques and a little fun to the home baker. Here are a few terms, tricks, and tools I'll be using.

Bonbons. Candy has many names: confections, pralines, sweets, chocolates, and, my favorite, bonbons. Translated from the French, it means "good goods," which always strikes me as the perfect name for chocolate candy.

Butter. European-style butter (such as Plugra) has a higher fat content than America's standard. Fat conducts flavor over the palate, so in this case, fat is good. Although the recipes in this book will work with American-style butter, I recommend using unsalted, European style, preferably from a dairy in your state.

Chocolate Choices. In many recipes, I've included "Chocolate Choices"—tips on which brands to consider for those particular recipes. These are just suggestions—the important thing is to have fun choosing chocolate.

Creaming Method for Cakes. Whipping butter and sugar together in a mixer (or by hand with a whisk), then adding eggs, then dry ingredients is a technique called "the creaming method," widely used in cake production. It makes for an airy, rich cake and is the basic technique for most of the cakes and cookies in this book. It's easy, just like making chocolate chip cookies. I don't mention it in the directions, but you'll notice its frequent use.

Fresh, Local Dairy Products. The best pastry chefs in the world insist on fresh ingredients for quality results, and you can insist on the same. Become a *locavore*— buy local milk, cream, butter, and eggs whenever possible. Unless you live near the equator, your chocolate never will be considered a local product because of its tropical origins. But the milk, cream, and eggs you need to make great desserts are easy to find at farmers' markets or health food shops. Also, organic dairy products are a good choice—they won't contain residue of pesticides, hormones, or additives.

Mise en Place. The French term for things "put in place" is a good one for the dessert baker to know. In some ways, it means read through your recipe, gather all your ingredients, measure them all out, *then* start mixing and baking. This saves you tons of trouble—you won't be halfway through a cake batter only to discover that you don't have any eggs. *Mise en place* is a philosophy of careful prep work.

Offset Spatula. The "L" shape of this long spatula allows flexibility for scraping chocolate and smoothing icings on cakes. I have twelve of these, but never feel like I have enough. Need a few? See Shopping Sources Guide, page 137.

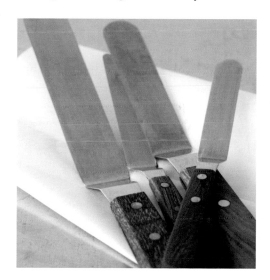

Salt. I use a lot of salt in my recipes because it enhances the flavor of chocolate. My measurements are based on coarse salts (like kosher and sea salt).

If you are using table salt (like Morton's Table Salt in the round paper container), use half of what is called for in my recipes. But I urge bakers to experiment with the different kinds of salt available in gourmet food stores because of the amazing range of subtle flavors. If you don't have time for such things, just grab a big box of kosher salt (Morton's also makes a good one) from the grocery store. If you have health issues like hypertension and have been advised to skip the salt, by all means do. The recipes will still hold up.

Stainless Steel Bowls. These rugged essentials are available at many large grocery stores and kitchen supply stores. You don't need fancy or heavy bowls, just several medium ones that you can plop over a pan of simmering water to melt your chocolate, then rinse and toss unceremoniously in the dishwasher.

Sugar and Alternative Sweeteners. Most of my recipes call for old-fashioned, granulated white sugar or brown sugar, sometimes quite a lot of both. You can explore the sweet treasures of health food stores, such as agave and malt syrups, forest honeys, and raw sugar if you prefer less processed sugar when I call for a cup of white.

Water Method. This technique for melting chocolate is based on the French technique *bain marie*, or water bath, which uses simmering water to heat a bowl of ingredients gently. Chefs often use the term to refer to all water-heating methods. For chocolate-melting purposes, place a heatproof bowl (a simple stainless steel one works best) of chocolate over a saucepan filled with about 3 inches of water. You want to keep the chocolate suspended above the water and keep the heat medium to low. The water becomes a gentle heat source. A double boiler will work for this job, too, but you don't need to make a special purchase. Once the water simmers (about 5 minutes), turn off the heat because the chocolate can overheat if left over a boiling pan. Then stir the chocolate occasionally until it is melted. (For more on melting chocolate, see page 24.) Another common water-heating method, used to make custard desserts such as cheesecake (page 90), involves a cake pan with batter placed in a larger pan. Water is added to the larger pan so that it reaches about halfway up the cake pan. This traditional water bath keeps the cake or custard baking slowly, moistly, and evenly.

Whipping Egg Whites. This is a love-hate challenge all bakers must tackle. How do you know if the eggs whites are whipped enough? Do they hold a soft peak? Medium peak? Stiff peak? What's a peak? Peaks indicate the structure achieved by whipping air into the protein molecules of egg whites at room temperature. If the whites are too cold or the mixer introduces foreign particles such as fats, the whites may not whip up at all (use a clean bowl and clean whisk). Soft peaks happen when you notice the egg whites transforming from yellow, stringy liquid to white foam. If you lift up your whisk from the bowl, you'll see the foamy egg whites droop off the whisk in a mound. That mound is called a soft peak. Keep going another minute or two, lift up your whisk, and you'll notice the egg whites form more of a defined, pointy peak and the whole batch looks thick and white. That's a medium peak. In just another minute or two of whipping, you'll reach stiff peaks, when the egg whites are at full volume, shiny, and decidedly hold a firm peak. If you beat them further, the protein that is holding the air breaks down and the egg whites become a puddle of lifeless goop. I like to take my egg whites off the mixer after they hit medium peak and beat them the rest of the way by hand. That prevents the danger of overbeating them. Always bake with extra eggs in the refrigerator so if you overbeat your egg whites, you can start over. Also, a dash of sugar at the beginning helps stabilize the egg whites. We use egg whites for meringues, icings, and cake batters.

> **bliss byte: chef's quote**
>
> Chocolate is a medium through which I narrate ideas. By exploring new cultures, movements, artists, religions, origins, and indigenous ingredients, a multi-sensory taste experience is created. Chocolate is a very powerful fruit.
>
> —Chocolatier Katrina Markoff, Vosges, Illinois

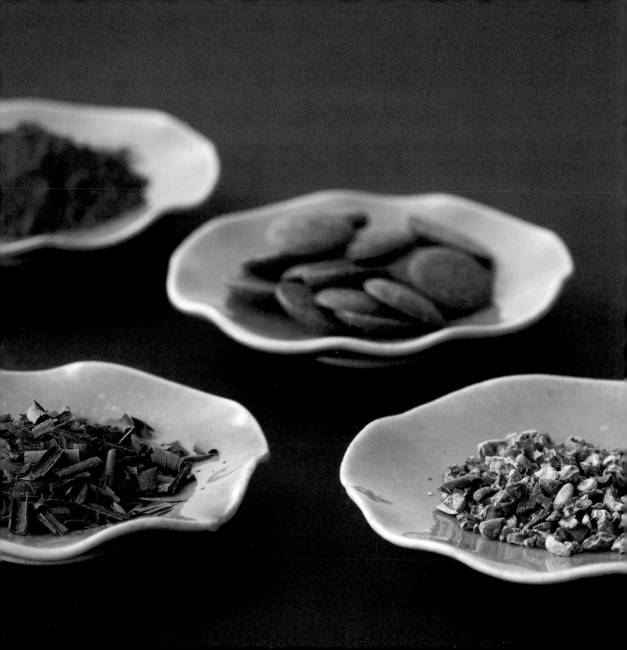

1 *good taste*

✦

EXPLORING YOUR
FAVORITE CHOCOLATES

The beauty of chocolate involves all of our senses. As we isolate and appreciate chocolate's effect on each of the five senses, we gain insight into its mysterious power.

your taste

You have good taste! Your chocolate preferences and pleasures are all your own, formed in childhood and developed over a lifetime. Like wine, chocolate is made from a fruit that has undergone fermentation, and its growing conditions affect its flavor. But unlike wine, you fall in love with chocolate when you are a baby, or as soon as some generous grown-up introduces you to the wonders of an overflowing candy bucket on Halloween. Maybe your first experience of chocolate was a birthday cake or a chocolate coin swap with other kids during the holidays. Maybe you were rewarded with chocolate for being a very good child instead of a bratty little monster! A growing stack of research suggests that these bright moments of childhood propel our positive associations with chocolate. So when we taste chocolate thoughtfully, we remember the chocolate we loved as children. Memory is a gateway into the arena of familiar chocolate flavors and the many more to be discovered.

Tasting chocolate as a connoisseur is simply learning how to appreciate and describe the depth of the flavors and feelings chocolate brings you. What you learn about great chocolate (also known as "couverture," "fine," or "premium" chocolate) will help you evaluate the difference between the best and the worst. (The worst is what the French call "junk chocolate," stripped of its natural cocoa butter and loaded with cheap additives such as palm oil or wax.) I can assure you it is possible to love the full range of chocolate, from the finest dark couvertures to the deliciously over-sugared, mass-produced, kid-friendly, melt-in-your-mouth junk we buy at the gas station.

Artisan foods and gourmet products have exploded in popularity over the last two decades, and now you can get great chocolate at supermarkets throughout the United States. At Publix in Atlanta, you'll find dark Lindt chocolate from Switzerland in the candy aisle next to big bags of Tootsie Rolls and Kit Kats. At any Trader Joe's on the West Coast, you'll find Valrhona Guanaja 70% cacao, a super-dark premium bar from France, at the checkout counter. Nestlé, famous for its old faithful Toll House Semi-Sweet Chocolate Morsels, now has an artisan line called Nestlé Chocolatier. Hershey's offers Cacao Reserve by Hershey's and Hershey's Whole Bean Chocolate, both much darker and less sweet than their everyday Hershey's Milk Chocolate bar. The widening availability and consumer enthusiasm for artisan chocolate is nothing less than an American chocolate revolution.

> ### bliss byte: storing chocolate
>
> Store chocolate in a dry spot at about 65°F. Keep it away from bright light, humidity, heat, and strong flavors, such as garlic, because it absorbs them.

what is artisan chocolate?

The term "artisan chocolate" describes premium chocolate made from high-quality beans in small batches. It differs from mass produced chocolate because it is made with more flavorful cacao beans and it is more carefully crafted. Two styles fall into the artisan category: "eating chocolate" (smooth, thin bars with no additives, centers, or decorations, and usually labels that include information about cacao percentages and the country of origin) and "bonbons" (bite-size chocolates filled with flavored centers or nuts or topped with decorations; these are also known as "candies," "pralines," or "confections"). Both types of artisan chocolates start with the highest-quality couverture, made from select seeds of cacao trees grown in tropical jungles around the world. Plantation workers hand-harvest cacao pods from the trees, split them, extract their seeds, carefully allow the seeds to ferment in big bins, then let the seeds or "beans" dry in the sun. From there, these beans are hulled, roasted, blended, and processed for distribution by primarily European and American companies.

You won't find many gourmet artisan bonbons in grocery stores because they are too delicate for mass distribution. You will find them, however, in small chocolate shops throughout Australia, the United States, Canada, Europe, and parts of Asia,

shopping! 10 great websites

Online shopping brings the world of chocolate to you. You can have the finest chocolates in the world delivered to your door. Avoid hot-weather delivery because chocolate melts so easily. Below are a few of my favorite shopping spots for everything from bonbons to bulk to bakeware.

Baker's Cash and Carry, www.bakerscandc.com.
Belgian Chocolate Online, www.chocolat.com.
Chef Shop, www.chefshop.com.
Chocolate Chocolate Chocolate Company, www.chocolate.com.
Chocolate Source, www.chocolatesource.com.
Chocosphere, www.chocosphere.com.
Gourmail, www.gourmail.com.
Surfas, www.surfasonline.com.
Whole Foods, www.wholefoods.com.
Worldwide Chocolate, www.worldwidechocolate.com.

most with online shopping sites as well. Great artisan bonbons start with great couverture, the very same you might choose as your favorite eating chocolate.

Maybe you like understated squares with minimal, natural decorations. Maybe you like old-fashioned gooey chocolates filled with marshmallow cream and covered with jimmies. Maybe you like colorful lineups of fanciful paintings, like those found in one of New York's best shops, Marie Belle (see listing, page 140). The design and flavor must work together, and every chocolatier seeks to achieve a pleasing balance. You get the final vote. The look must win your eyes, and the flavor must win your heart.

have a chocolate tasting

The best way to appreciate artisan chocolates and the range of flavors now available is to prepare a chocolate tasting for yourself (and perhaps a few friends). In the business, this is called a "focused chocolate tasting." By choosing your chocolates and textures thoughtfully, you are continuing the work of the chocolate growers, producers, and artisans who brought the best of their craft to you. Chocolate comes in four main categories: dark chocolate, milk chocolate, white chocolate, and cocoa powder. While cocoa powder has many great culinary uses, in tasting sessions it is always dry and bitter, so it is not very interesting to evaluate. Focus on the other three.

Dark Chocolate. Dark chocolate presents the cleanest, most powerful flavors, so you'll want to include it in your tasting. Even if you are a loyal milk chocolate lover, buy at least three dark chocolate bars with similar compositions. Dark chocolate can be "unsweetened," which is very bitter, with no sugar at all; "bittersweet," which combines bitter and sweet flavors, often in the 70% cacao range; or "semisweet," which is the sweetest of the darks, often in the 60% cacao range. Look for brands with no nuts or fillings, such as Green & Black's, Lindt, Newman's Own, Hershey's, Scharffen Berger, or Valrhona.

Milk Chocolate. Milk chocolate starts out as dark chocolate and is then processed with more sugar and milk powder (or combination of powder and liquid known as "milk crumb"). Good milk chocolate is 38 to 50% cacao; the rest sugar and milk powder. Each manufacturer has a different recipe for the proportions. Again, for the purpose of taste comparison, look for brands with no nuts or fillings, such as Lindt, Cadbury, Endangered Species, Scharffen Berger, Green & Black's, Hershey's, or Chocolove.

White Chocolate. White chocolate is not really chocolate. It is cocoa butter, sugar, and milk powder, plus a few flavorings. Because cocoa butter comes from the cocoa bean, white chocolate has a mild flavor of chocolate, without any of the strength or power. It is often used in desserts and confectionary as an accent to darker chocolates. Look for white chocolate bars with no nuts or additives. Try Lindt, Nestlé, El Rey, or Ghirardelli.

defining flavors

The words to describe chocolate's flavors ("descriptors") are much like those used for wine: "bouquet," "notes," "undertones," and "finish." Within chocolate's deep flavors lie hints of other flavors. These are the specific "flavor notes" you might describe, like plums, caramel, grass, or sour cherries. Dark artisan chocolate is often described as "fruity," "earthy," "bitter," or "acidic." If you notice fruit-like notes as you taste a piece of dark chocolate, the flavor may remind you of raspberries. Or it may remind you of raisins. Or it may taste like raspberries, then raisins. No one suggests that the chocolate actually contains these fruits; we're talking only about similar flavor notes. By describing these subtle distinctions, you are exercising your skill as a chocolate taster.

For many, the powerful complexity of dark chocolate is more sophisticated than sweeter, creamier milk chocolate. Dark chocolate is chocolate, and milk chocolate is a sugary confection, connoisseurs might say. Yet the world is full of milk chocolate lovers, and sales of milk chocolate compose 70 percent of the chocolate business world-wide. Some of the most careful discriminators of chocolate flavors enjoy the complementary relationship between the bitter and the sweet. *Cook's Illustrated* magazine ran a survey of two hundred food editors around the United States to determine the most popular premium chocolate, and surprisingly, it was not esteemed brands from

techniques for tasting

- Borrow the "flight" technique from wine tasting so that you compare flavors of similarly sweetened chocolates. Compare small pieces of dark to dark, milk to milk, white to white. Also consider comparing chocolates with similar percentages of cacao (70% cacao with others in that range, 50% cacao with others in *that* range).

- Start with dark chocolate comparisons, take a break, then move up to milk chocolate. Take another break, and then finish with white chocolate. Always move from dark to light to keep the palate free of dairy and sugar.

- Let the chocolate melt on the tongue, then move it to the back teeth, give it three bites, move it all around the mouth, then allow it to rest and melt more. Notice how the flavors change and develop.

- Enjoy the "long finish" of great chocolate—the lingering flavors left on the palate are among the strongest and most telling.

- Use water to cleanse the palate between tastes.

- Write descriptors on notepads as the chocolate melts in your mouth, since it is hard to savor and speak at the same time. Think about what flavors or scents the chocolate evokes, such as honey, raspberries, earth, or mushrooms. Then take a moment to compare your descriptors with those of others in your group. You'll probably find some common ground.

bliss byte: mesoamerica

The ancient cultural world of what is now southern Mexico and Central America before the Spanish conquistadores arrived in 1508 is Mesoamerica, where cacao trees and chocolate were first cultivated. The traditions of four main tribes—the Olmec, the Maya, the Toltec, and the Aztec (about 1500 B.C.E. to 1508 C.E.)—include chocolate as a spicy drink, a form of currency, and/or a religious sacrament. We won't get to explore all the glorious representations of chocolate in Mesoamerican mythologies, art, ceramics, trading patterns, and religions because if we did, there would be no room in this book for cake and cookie recipes! For fascinating reading on the use of chocolate in these cultures, see "Great Books on Chocolate History," page 27.

Europe, such as Valrhona or Amedei. It was San Francisco's own Ghirardelli, a sweet dark from their premium line. One of the great values of chocolate tasting is there is no right or wrong. We don't need to judge, only to explore.

You might see a buffet of exotic chocolate bars at your gourmet grocers: Tanzania (83% cacao) next to Ecuador (82% cacao) or a single-estate Arriba (78% cacao). Which is better? "The single-origin movement is driven by marketing," says Peter Greweling, professor of baking and pastry at the prestigious Culinary Institute of America and author of *Chocolate and Confections* (see "Great Books of Chocolate Recipes," page 20). "No question that varieties from different regions taste different. It's the terroir, and it is interesting. But skillful blends of different cacaos—not just single origin—bring more complexity to chocolate." His opinion is shared by many fine couverture makers. "Try them all," he concludes happily. Valrhona makes irresistible tasting packages, as does Pralus in Belgium, and Scharffen Berger, Hershey's, and Vosges Haut-Chocolat in the United States.

fragrance and flavor

You know the smell I mean. You put the pan of brownies in the oven at 2:17 P.M. on a Saturday afternoon and around 2:53 P.M. your kids zoom into the kitchen, searching the countertops for the hot pan. You lured them with chocolate's fragrance, an aroma that triggers memories, hunger, and joy.

Scientists use the word "flavor" to mean three components of the sensory properties of food: basic tastes (sweet, salty, sour, and bitter), smell (aroma, the most complex of the components), and something called "chemical feeling factors" (such as the way cinnamon burns, the way mint cools). Chocolate's powerful aroma is released by heat. So when rising heat from a warm, dark brownie travels through the nose and is followed by a big gooey bite that covers all the taste buds and receptors with its sweet, molten chocolateyness . . . that is about as complete a flavor experience as you can have.

What brand should you use for the optimum brownie? You'll want a strong, fragrant one, which is something to seek at your chocolate tasting. After you've translated the messages on the label, a quick sniff will send some flavor information your way. Is it strong? Mild? Fruity? Sour? Burned? Does it evoke childhood memories, or is it richer than what you may have known in your early chocolate days? Your sense of smell and your sense of taste are a team effort.

Chances are your chocolate tasting will involve small pieces of cool or room temperature chocolate. But if you've got the time, consider sampling a melted chocolate flight to observe how powerful the warm aromas can be. In my opinion, this is the secret beauty of the classic kid favorite, s'mores. Sure, the squishy marshmallow is important, but it is the fragrance, texture, and sweetness of pure melted chocolate that take center stage on the graham cracker. One of America's best chocolatiers,

label language 101

Fine chocolate is labeled with information about its origin and content. Here are some common phrases and translations.

Baking Chocolate. American term for unsweetened chocolate, usually the Baker's brand.

Bean to Bar. Refers to chocolate makers who include the process of roasting, grinding, and seasoning chocolate, as opposed to working with couverture made by specialists such as Barry Callebaut or Valrhona.

Cacao. Refers to ground beans from cacao trees, also known as "cocoa liquor" or "cocoa mass." "Cacao" generally refers to the trees and their products; "cocoa" refers to those products as they move through the chocolate-making process. On a label, "72% cacao" indicates a high percentage of cocoa mass as opposed to additives.

Cocoa Nibs. Pure cocoa beans that have been fermented, hulled, roasted, and cracked but not ground into a paste. They have a nutlike crunch.

Cocoa Powder or Cocoa. Pure cocoa solids pressed from cacao beans with cocoa butter removed. It may or may not have been treated with alkali to improve balance. Cocoa without alkali is generally healthier (depending on the roasting temperatures) and reddish in color; cocoa with alkali is smoother and darker.

Country of Origin. Refers to the specific country in the growing region.

Grand Cru. Indicates that beans were derived from one select cacao plantation.

72% Cacao. A dark bittersweet chocolate, 72 percent of which is crushed cacao beans (cocoa mass), the other 18 percent mostly sugar. These percentages range from the 60s to the 80s for dark chocolate. High percentages suggest quality but do not guarantee it since the quality of the beans matters most.

Single Estate. Beans were derived from one select cacao plantation.

62% Cacao. A semisweet dark chocolate with more sugar and other ingredients. Quality milk chocolate or sweet dark chocolates fall in the range of 40 to 50 percent cacao.

Soy Lecithin. An emulsifier made from soy beans.

Michael Recchiuti of San Francisco, includes a gourmet interpretation of s'mores in his product line. It is a best-seller.

touching chocolate

Chocolate's one-of-a-kind texture comes from its one-of-a-kind fat: cocoa butter. All chocolate except for cocoa powder contains cocoa butter, which conducts all the flavor-rich chocolate solids that move over your taste buds. Most of the compounds in cocoa butter melt around 91°F. You, as a healthy human being, are at 98°F. Every time cocoa butter touches you, it melts. This is a lovely quality in any friend or food, but it also contributes to chocolate's biggest production problem: separation. Melted cocoa butter (fat) pulls away from cocoa solids (proteins and carbs) as it solidifies and leaves two unattached and unappealing substances. The cocoa butter is grey and greasy, the cocoa solids are dry and crumbly. This explains why chocolate was used in liquid form for centuries—warm, liquefied chocolate was easier for people to keep together. Solid, block chocolate was invented much later in England in 1866, and the process known as chocolate "tempering" became standard. Tempering brings the fats and solids together for keeps and allows for the many uses we know today (see "Techniques for Tempering," page 37). All modern chocolate bars (artisan or otherwise) have been tempered at the factory—one of many processes that bring them from bean to bar. All this chemistry results in the interplay between texture and taste known as "mouthfeel." Chocolate, when all its parts are harmoniously blended, has a perfectly smooth mouthfeel. This contributes to chocolate's long-term status on lists of sexy foods. The melting texture, the evolving flavors, the thickness, bitterness, and sweetness together give chocolate its unique sensuality. This moment of pleasure is always worth noticing as you taste chocolate.

listening to chocolate

Snap! It's the sound a thin, premium dark chocolate bar makes when you break off that first piece to sample. It's also the sound dark chocolate makes when you bite it. To a lesser degree, it is the sound that any chocolate candy makes as you break through the shell and into the creamy center. Snap, like shine (see below), is an indicator of well-made, well-tempered chocolate.

You won't get as dramatic a snap from milk or white chocolate, since the volume of other ingredients (sugar and dairy) reduces the amount of cocoa solids. But you'll notice a definite snappy something. (You will also notice a lack of snap if you come across untempered chocolate, which you might if yours has melted and resolidified.) Break a few pieces with your friends as you gather for your chocolate tasting. Hearing a good snap creates anticipation for a good chocolate flavor.

behold, great chocolate!

Artisan chocolatiers make fashion statements. A chocolatier's window might showcase the dark shine of bonbons made with 72% cacao dark chocolate nestled next to the tan hues of milk chocolate, accented by the drama of pink peppercorns or pistachio pieces. When you gaze into an artisan chocolatier's window, you should see a show of shiny coats and subtle decorations that no machine could ever approximate. You might like small dark squares with just a spray of sea salt on top. Or you might prefer elaborately molded seashells, prisms, or voluptuous dark hearts trimmed with gold. The wide-ranging creative workmanship of today's top chocolatiers has set new standards for the chocolate industry and given the chocolate connoisseur more choices than ever.

All great artisan chocolates have one visual thing in common: a shiny surface. Shine indicates that the chocolate is well tempered and well balanced. It should have no grey streaks (known as "fat bloom"), no dewey spots (known as "sugar bloom"), no clumpy corners, no broken shells. Beyond these simple common denominators, finished chocolate products are made beautiful by the imaginations and skilled hands of artisan chocolatiers.

great websites for info, recipes, and blogs

www.barry-callebaut.com. Descriptions of the growing regions, product lines, culinary applications, and professional education.

www.carolebloom.com. A site from a chocolate cookbook author with European techniques and American know-how.

www.chocomap.com. A Canadian chocolatier and educator connects chocolate enthusiasts with quality shops in far-flung areas.

www.epicurious.com. A recipe site run by the good people of *Bon Appétit* magazine.

www.fieldmuseum.org/chocolate. The Field Museum in Chicago sponsored an exhibit chronicling chocolate's history, including paintings of the chocolate-drinking aristocracy.

www.foodnetwork.com. Search for recipes and TV shows featuring chocolate.

www.70percent.com. An informational site and blog; those with serious questions and big opinions should spend some time here.

www.thechocolatelife.com. A social networking group featuring discussions between fellow enthusiasts, bloggers, and experts, plus announcements about culinary events.

www.valrhona.com. A site that will explain to you what makes great chocolate great.

www.worldcocoafoundation.com. This site focuses on the growing regions, offering news, conferences, and initiatives to help those involved with cacao farming around the world.

great books of chocolate recipes

All About Chocolate by Carole Bloom. Classic recipes for desserts like brownies and German chocolate cake and also resources for equipment and chocolate travel.

Cocolat: Extraordinary Chocolate Desserts by Alice Medrich. Medrich delights her readers with wisdom and clarity, just as she delighted the loyal customers of her San Francisco dessert shops, Cocolat.

The Chocolate Bible: The Definitive Sourcebook by Christian Tuebner et al. This book inspires on all levels. It is big; its pictures are beautiful; its classic cakes are moist and rich; its confections are wildly pretty; its recipes are professional but approachable.

Chocolate and Confections: Formula, Theory, and Technique for the Artisan Confectioner by Peter Greweling. A professor of baking and pastry at the Culinary Institute of America gives specific techniques for mastering confections.

Chocolate Passion: Recipes and Inspiration from the Kitchens of Chocolatier Magazine by Tish Boyle and Tim Moriarty. This book offers the delicious quality you'd expect from the editors of the magazine now called *Dessert Professional*.

Dessert Circus by Jacques Torres. Torres speaks to the home craftsperson in a way that informs and encourages mastery over the sometimes difficult skills of chocolate work.

The Essence of Chocolate: Recipes for Baking and Cooking with Fine Chocolate by John Scharffenberger and Robert Steinberg. This dramatic story of how Dr. Robert Steinberg moved from a cancer diagnosis to establishing the premier chocolate-making company in the country is great reading, plus the book contains dessert recipe treasures.

Fine Chocolate, Great Experiences by Jean-Pierre Wybauw. A revered chocolate professional delights in the chemistry of chocolate, and his recipes provide great attention to detail.

The Great Book of Chocolate by David Lebovitz. This informative book by Lebovitz, who conducts culinary tours of Parisian chocolate shops, is jaunty and fun to read.

Maida Heatter's Book of Great Chocolate Desserts by Maida Heatter. Most bakers have had someone they love teach them how. Because of this chocolate cookbook and many others, Maida Heatter is America's most beloved baking teacher.

the chocolate-tasting finale

I like to close my chocolate tastings by presenting many of my favorite artisan bonbons, which is a splurge. I scheme, shop online, and drive embarrassing distances to collect a wide range of tantalizing chocolates for contrast in style and flavor. I include hand-made confections and beautiful bonbons from great chocolatiers (in flavors like bourbon ganache, passion fruit, sesame nougat, and orange cardamom) lined up on white plates. For a chocolate tasting connected to a dinner party with friends, I conduct the chocolate tasting, serve dinner (maybe a sandwich bar with hams and cheeses and fresh greens), then present a very chocolate cake made with one of the chocolates considered in the session. I serve hot chocolate and coffee in addition to the array of bonbons. My goal is to celebrate all the senses with my guests. Your tasting can conclude with this kind of finale, or it can end with a quiet flight of bold red wines, sliced fruit, and more of your favorite chocolates.

bliss byte: chocolate and wine pairings

Dark Chocolate and Red Wine. Contrast and compare the red fruit notes found in dark chocolate and fruity reds such as pinot noir, syrah, and zinfandel.

Milk Chocolate and Champagne. Dry white wines like brut Champagne, chardonnay, and Chablis balance the sweetness of milk chocolate. Celebrate!

sensuous recipes: from bonbons to fondue

These recipes celebrate the sensuous wonders of chocolate. While some appeal more to smell, some to taste, and some to touch, they should all appeal to the appreciative nature of a chocolate lover.

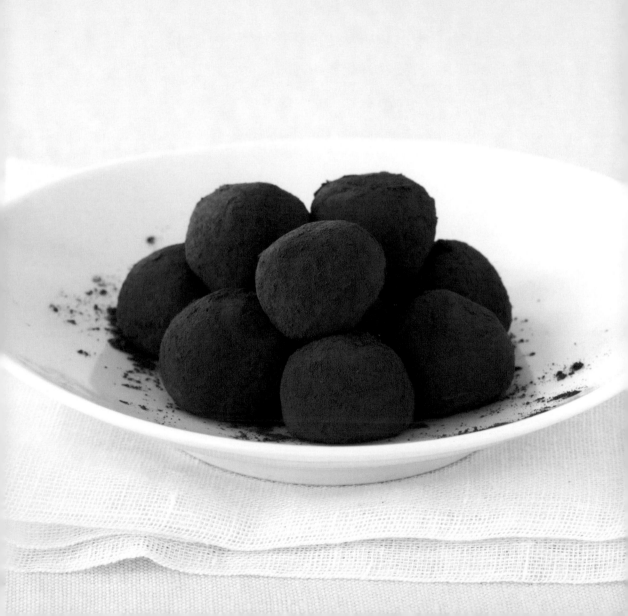

artisan caramel bonbons

Handmade caramel is sophisticated and soothingly sweet, especially when combined with the bold flavors of artisan chocolate. You can also dip these bonbons in tempered chocolate before you dust them to create chocolate caramel truffles. **Makes about 30 truffles**

Prepare a bowl of ice water and set aside. Combine the sugar, water, and corn syrup in a heavy pan. Stir gently until all the sugar is wet, and make sure no sugar crystals are on the sides of the pan. Place over medium heat—no stirring—and allow the mixture to boil for about 10 minutes. You can cover the pan for a few minutes as it boils, which will wash away any unwanted sugar crystals on the sides. You'll start to see a light amber color form around the edges of the sugar. Continue boiling until the mixture is the color of honey or maple syrup. This is now caramel, so be careful because it is very hot!

Turn off the heat and plunge the saucepan into the ice water to "shock" the sugar and stop it from cooking. Place the pot on a heatproof surface, add the butter, then the cream, vanilla, and salt. It will steam and bubble up. Stir it together, and once the mixture has cooled off (about 10 minutes), add the dark and milk chocolates and stir until mixed. If the caramel sticks to the bottom of the pan, return the pot to the burner and stir over very low heat.

Transfer this mixture to a bowl and allow it to cool and firm up in the refrigerator for about 30 minutes. With a melon baller or sturdy spoon, scoop out as many balls as you need (any unused portion can be reheated and used as a sauce over ice cream). Roll them between your palms to achieve a round shape. Refrigerate them for about 30 minutes, then dust them with cocoa powder and serve.

Chocolate Choices

Green & Black's or Michel Cluizel dark chocolate, Scharffen Berger milk chocolate

2 cups sugar

1/4 cup water

1/4 cup light corn syrup

6 tablespoons (3/4 stick) unsalted butter

1/2 cup heavy cream

1 teaspoon vanilla extract

2 teaspoons kosher salt

8 ounces dark chocolate (70% cacao or higher), finely chopped

4 ounces milk chocolate, finely chopped

2 ounces unsweetened cocoa powder, for dusting

chopping and melting chocolate

Why do so many recipes call for chocolate to be "finely chopped"? Chocolate melts more uniformly when it is chopped into very small pieces. Thin bars or disks of couverture (also known as "callets") are easy to chop up. Chocolate in bulk, however, is usually a giant, rock-hard, and impossibly thick block. This big block melts in your hands when you pick it up. If you wrestle it down into a bowl to melt, you'll probably wind up with the edges completely melted and the center completely solid. Instead, while it is still in its original wrapper, hold one end of the package firmly and give it a couple of whacks with a hammer to break it into manageable pieces to chop. From there, a few more tricks:

1. Use a serrated knife (bread knife). This gives you more traction against the chocolate and also works like a grate.

2. Wear bicycle gloves. Yes, you'll look like a geek, but the padded palms, open finger-tips, and washability are perfect for chocolate work.

3. Take one of the broken chunks of chocolate and chop it from corner to corner. In other words, don't start in the middle because you'll get more resistance.

4. Try a "chocolate chipper." This is a gadget similar to an ice pick available in gourmet kitchenware stores.

Two words when it comes to chocolate melting: *low* and *slow*. Chocolate melts easily, which is great, but it also burns easily, so you have to melt it carefully—over low heat and slowly. Here are the three best ways:

1. Water method. See page 4.

2. Low oven. If you have an oven with a pilot light, the inside of the oven is probably about 100°F. Place the chocolate in a heatproof bowl or pie pan and it will melt slowly. If you do turn on the heat, use the lowest setting and keep an eye on it. Anything above 120°F is too hot for chocolate.

3. Microwave. It's risky. It's frowned upon in many chocolate circles. But it is certainly pos-sible to melt chocolate using a microwave oven effectively if you remember: *low* and

slow. Place the chocolate in a Pyrex cup, bowl, or pie plate and program the microwave for 30 seconds on low heat. Then take the chocolate out, stir it, and put it back in for another 30 seconds. You'll need to repeat this process three or four times. This slightly tedious approach will assure you that you don't burn the chocolate, which is very easy to do in general and especially easy to do in a microwave oven.

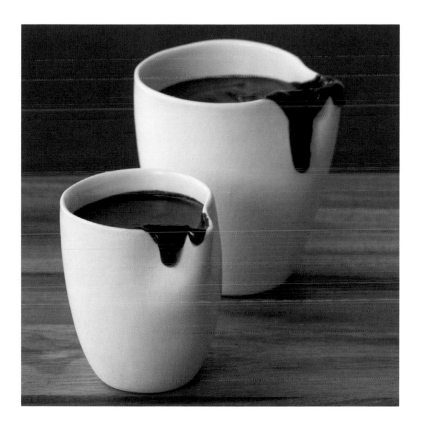

breakfast-in-bed pound cake

A slice of this chocolate-ribboned cake served on a tray with a cup of hot cocoa, a glass of chilled juice, and a boiled egg, accompanied by a newspaper and a little flower in a vase, will please the soul of any chocolate lover lying in bed. Not so sure? Add a chocolate glaze (see Glaze of the Gods, page 118) and you'll be guaranteed entry into the boudoir of chocolate heaven. **Makes 1 (9-inch) cake**

2 cups cake flour

1 teaspoon baking powder

1 1/2 teaspoons kosher salt

1/2 cup sour cream

1/2 cup whole or 2% milk

1 tablespoon vanilla extract

1 cup (2 sticks) cold unsalted butter, cut into small pieces

1 1/4 cups sugar

4 large eggs, at room temperature

3 ounces dark chocolate (preferably semisweet), melted

2 tablespoons light corn syrup

1 tablespoon water

Preheat the oven to 350°F. Generously grease a Bundt or loaf pan (about 4 inches tall and 9 inches in diameter).

Sift together the cake flour, baking powder, and salt and set aside. In a different bowl, combine the sour cream, milk, and vanilla extract and set aside.

In the bowl of an electric mixer fitted with the paddle attachment, cream the butter on low speed for several minutes. Change to the whisk attachment, slowly add the sugar, then mix at medium-high speed for a few more minutes, until this mixture is light and fluffy. Turn the mixer to low and add the eggs, one at a time, beating after each one until incorporated. Stop the mixer and add half of the flour mixture, then mix slowly. Next, add half of the sour cream mixture and mix slowly. Repeat this process so that all the flour and sour cream mixtures are incorporated. You'll now have a bowl of vanilla batter.

Pour one-third of the vanilla batter into a small bowl. Add the melted chocolate, corn syrup, and water and stir until smooth. This becomes your "chocolate batter."

Pour the vanilla batter into the prepared pan. Pour the chocolate batter over the vanilla batter. Use the tip of a spatula to swirl the chocolate batter lightly through the vanilla batter. Another way to achieve the marble effect is to put both batters in pastry bags and squeeze them into the pan in a random marbled pattern.

Bake for 40 minutes, or until the top of the cake is springy and a toothpick inserted in the center comes out clean. When the cake is done, remove it from the oven and allow it to cool completely in the pan on a rack. Once it is cool, invert the pan and allow the cake to gently fall onto a cake plate.

great books on chocolate history

Chocolate: An Illustrated History by Marcia and Frederic Morton. Charming prose and solid scholarship.

Chocolate: History, Culture, and Heritage by Louis E. Grivetti. An in-depth chocolate history project from the University of California, Davis, and Mars, Inc.

Chocolate in Mesoamerica edited by Cameron L. McNeil. A thorough analysis of artifacts and culture.

The New Taste of Chocolate by Maricel E. Presilla. Chef, author, and historian, Presilla explains how to taste chocolate in thoughtful, commonsense language. The book conveys her deep knowledge of Venezuelan cacao farming and chocolate making.

The Temptation of Chocolate by Jacques Mercer. A journey through the world of chocolate from Neuhaus, inventors of the praline.

The True History of Chocolate by Sophie D. Coe and Michael D. Coe. You'll find this book referenced more than any contemporary book on chocolate history. Both scholarly and entertaining, it covers everything from trees to Mesoamericans to European royal courts.

heart and soul hot cocoa

This rich cocoa warms the heart and soul like no other. After you've served the cocoa, the leftover amount makes a good base for chilly chocolate milk the next day. Store it in the refrigerator and just splash in cold, fresh milk to lighten it up. **Makes 6 to 8 servings**

Chocolate Choices

Cocoa powders to consider are E. Guittard, Droste, Hershey's, Scharffen Berger, or—by far my favorite—Valrhona.

3/4 cup sugar, or more

1/2 cup unsweetened alkalized or dutched cocoa powder, or more to taste

4 cups whole milk

1/2 cup heavy cream

2 tablespoons malt syrup (optional)

1 tablespoon vanilla extract

1/2 teaspoon kosher salt

Artisan marshmallows or whipped cream (optional)

Mix the sugar and cocoa together in a small bowl and set aside. Combine the milk, cream, and malt syrup in a big saucepan over medium heat. As the milk starts to warm up, scoop up about a cup of it and slowly whisk it into the sugar and cocoa mixture to form a paste. Add the paste to the saucepan and whisk until incorporated. Add the vanilla and salt. Adjust the flavors to taste. Continue heating until it is hot but not boiling. Use a ladle to scoop out servings into a mug. Serve with artisan marshmallows or a dollop of whipped cream.

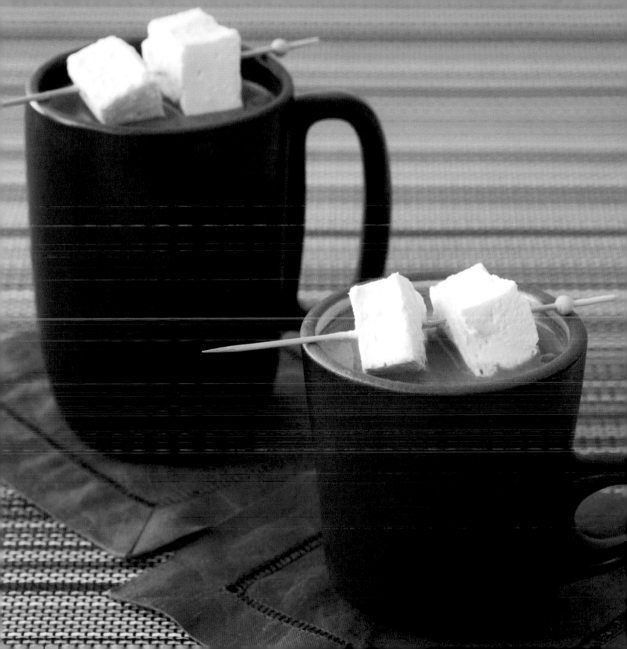

chocolate chip custard tart

This tart combines the pleasures of a rich chocolate custard with the crunchy appeal of a chocolate chip cookie. As with most pies and tarts, you have two steps: the crust and the filling. Collect the ingredients for both the crust dough and the filling, but make the dough first. As it chills, prepare the filling. **Makes 1 (9 or 10-inch) tart**

Chocolate Choices

For the crust: E. Guittard or Nestlé Chocolatier chocolate chips
For the custard: Felchlin Cru Sauvage or Scharffen Berger dark chocolate and Cadbury milk chocolate

Crust

3/4 cup (1 1/2 sticks) unsalted cold butter

1/2 cup sugar

3/4 cup firmly packed light brown sugar

2 large eggs

1 1/2 cups all-purpose flour

1 tablespoon vanilla extract

1 teaspoon kosher salt

12 ounces chocolate chips or dark chocolate, chopped into bite-size chunks

1/2 cup broken pecans (optional)

To make the crust dough, cream the butter in the bowl of an electric mixer fitted with the paddle attachment at medium speed for a minute or two. Stop the mixer and switch to the whisk attachment. Slowly add the sugars and mix at medium speed until light and fluffy, then add the eggs, one at a time, mixing until incorporated after each addition. Add the flour slowly, then the vanilla, salt, chocolate chips, and nuts, mixing until blended. Cover and chill for at least 20 minutes.

Lightly flour a cool rolling surface such as a marble tabletop. No marble tabletop? Just flip over a baking sheet, and flour it generously or lightly flour a big piece of parchment paper or silicone baking mat. Place the dough on the floured surface, lightly flour the top, and roll it with a rolling pin until just under 1/2 inch thick. No rolling pin? Flatten the dough as thinly as you can with your hands. Maneuver the flattened dough into a 9 or 10-inch tart or pie pan. One way to do this is to lift under the dough with a big spatula and slip the pan under the dough. Don't worry if the dough breaks—you can pinch it back together. Once the dough is in the pan, smooth it out and flatten it with your hands and press it against the edges of the tart pan. Use scissors to trim any excess pieces that hang over the sides (you can save these scraps and bake them as cookies later). Cover the dough with plastic wrap or aluminum foil and return it to the refrigerator.

Preheat oven to 300°F. To make the filling, melt the dark and milk chocolates and butter together in a stainless steel bowl over a saucepan of simmering water.

In a medium bowl, whisk together the eggs, brown sugar, salt, and vanilla extract and set aside. In a small saucepan, heat the milk and cream to a scald. Slowly add the milk mixture into the egg mixture while stirring briskly. Once the mixture is smooth, stir in the chocolate mixture and let cool to close to room temperature. This is your custard.

Remove the tart pan from the refrigerator, unwrap it, and put it on a baking sheet. Carefully pour the custard into the tart shell. Place the full tart pan into the hot oven. Take a standard cake pan and fill it halfway up with room temperature water. Place that pan next to the sheet pan in the oven to provide extra moisture for the tart while it bakes. Bake about 40 minutes. You'll see the cookie shell firm up and turn golden brown, and if you shake the pan a little you'll notice the custard moves as a solid, not a liquid. If it still wiggles like a liquid, give it another 5 minutes and try again. When the cookie is golden brown and the center is solid, remove the pan from the oven. Allow to cool to room temperature, then chill in the refrigerator for at least an hour. Serve cold or at room temperature. Slice with a big knife or pie cutter, and top each slice with a small scoop of whipped cream.

Filling

3 ounces dark chocolate, finely chopped

2 ounces milk chocolate, finely chopped

1/4 cup (1/2 stick) unsalted butter

2 large eggs at room temperature

2 heaping tablespoons light brown sugar

1 teaspoon kosher or coarse salt

1 teaspoon vanilla extract

1/2 cup milk at room temperature

1/2 cup heavy cream at room temperature

1 cup cream, whipped (optional)

deepest, darkest fudge brownies

No apologies here. These are dense and decadent. You'll want to use a strong dark chocolate—something that stands up to the richness of great butter, fresh eggs, and a lot of sugar. **Makes about 20 (2-inch square) brownies**

Chocolate Choices

Scharffen Berger, Domori, Lindt, or Trader Joe's Pound Plus 72% dark chocolate

1 1/2 cups all-purpose flour

2 tablespoons unsweetened cocoa powder

1 teaspoon kosher salt

8 ounces dark chocolate, finely chopped

1 cup (2 sticks) butter (preferably unsalted European style, such as Plugra)

5 large eggs

1 tablespoon vanilla extract

1 tablespoon strong brewed coffee or espresso

2 1/2 cups sugar

1 cup broken walnuts or pecans

Sifted confectioners' sugar, to dust

Preheat the oven to 350°F. Prepare a standard (13 by 9-inch) brownie pan by lining it with a sheet of parchment paper or lightly spraying the pan with cooking spray.

Sift together the flour, cocoa powder, and salt in a bowl, stir, then set aside.

Place the chocolate and butter together in a stainless steel bowl over a saucepan of simmering water and allow them to melt together.

In the bowl of an electric mixer fitted with the wire whip attachment, combine the eggs, vanilla, and coffee and mix on low speed until blended. Add half of the sugar, then mix on high. As the mixture becomes lighter, stop the mixer and add the remaining sugar. Whip until the mixture is smooth. Remove the bowl from the mixer and stir in the melted chocolate and butter. Add half the flour, fold in by hand, then add the rest of the flour and continue folding. Finally, fold in the nuts. Fold until the batter is smooth. Pour the batter into the prepared pan.

Bake for about 30 minutes. The cake will still be gooey in the center; the top and sides should be crispy. Allow the brownies to cool on a rack in the pan for about 30 minutes. Place the pan in the refrigerator for about an hour if possible to condense the moisture inside. Remove the pan from the refrigerator. Take a paring knife and run it around the sides of the pan, loosening the cake from the pan. Cover it with a sheet pan or large cutting board covered with parchment paper and flip it, allowing the brownie cake to gently fall onto the parchment paper. The cake will be upside down. Remove the baking pan, remove the parchment paper it baked on, then place a large cutting board over the cake, and flip it back over. Your cake is now right side up. You can slice the brownies into square or triangle shapes and dust with confectioners' sugar.

chocolate in the arts: poetry

No sooner have you swallowed a generous
    mouthful
This pearl, this jewel, this marvelous potion
    of the Americas
It has barely begun to melt within you
Yet it cleanses you and purifies you
Of all bitterness and all mortal cares.
Seeping into your arteries and your veins
In a beauteous concoction of vermillion sauce,
By its pleasant and free flow, it recalls
The torrid heat of the sun.

—Henry Stubbes, England, 1662

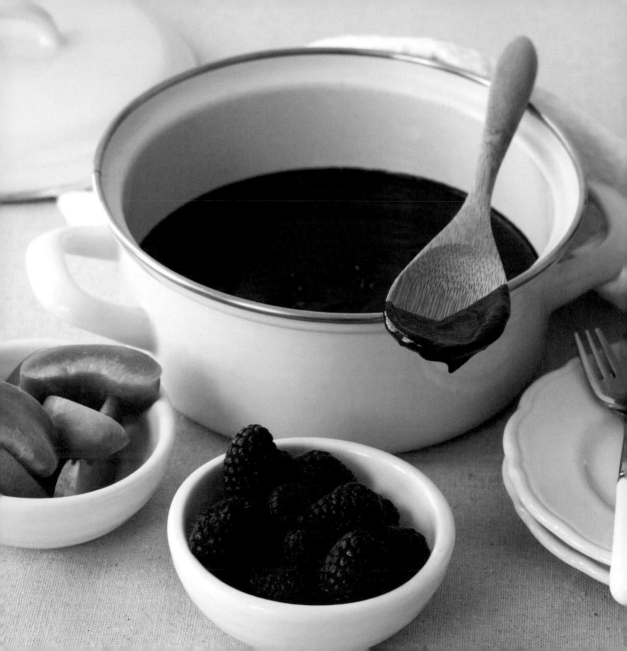

melting moment chocolate fondue

At the moment chocolate melts together with cream, butter, and vanilla, the senses awaken. Taste and texture are the stars of this warm, drippy dessert. For a gourmet add-on, make your own cookies to dip in the fondue. **Makes about 2 cups fondue**

Combine all the ingredients in a stainless steel bowl over a saucepan of simmering water. Keep the heat low and stir occasionally until the chocolate melts and the mixture is smooth and shiny. Then transfer to a fondue pot or serving bowl that can be suspended over heat (think ovenproof ceramic suspended over a candle). Serve with sliced seasonal fruit.

Chocolate Choices

Endangered Species or Cacao Barry Origins dark chocolate, such as Tanzanie, and Valrhona milk chocolate

8 ounces dark chocolate, finely chopped

2 ounces milk chocolate

1 cup heavy cream

1/4 cup (1/2 stick) unsalted butter

1 tablespoon light corn syrup

2 tablespoons cognac (optional; if you use less cognac, use a little more cream)

1 tablespoon vanilla extract

Pinch of kosher salt

fudgey hearts of darkness

This is a classic fudge with the full flavors of fine chocolate and cooked cream. You'll need a small, heart-shaped cookie cutter. Otherwise, you can cut it into simple squares or triangle shapes. **Makes about 20 (1-inch) squares**

Chocolate Choices

Theo Chocolate, Newman's Own, Climate Change, E. Guittard, or Lindt dark chocolate

1 1/2 cups Milk Chocolate Dulce de Leche (page 89) or 1 (14-ounce) can sweetened condensed milk

1 cup sugar

2 tablespoons unsalted butter

8 ounces dark chocolate, finely chopped

1 tablespoon vanilla extract

1 teaspoon salt

1/2 cup roasted walnuts, broken

Grease a 9-inch pan (square or round).

Combine the dulce de leche, sugar, and butter in a heavy saucepan over medium heat. Bring to a boil and continue cooking for about 5 minutes, or until you hit 235°F on a digital or candy thermometer. Take the pan off the heat and fold in the chocolate, vanilla, salt, and walnuts. Stir vigorously for several minutes, until the mixture is very smooth, then pour into the prepared pan.

Allow the mixture to set, about 30 minutes. Slice with a small heart-shaped cookie cutter. This fudge is very rich, so if you can't find a small heart-shaped cookie cutter, use a paring knife to cut out small, uniform heart shapes. Keep a bowl of hot water and a damp cloth nearby to clean the cutter or knife after each cut. If the fudge is too soft to cut easily, chill it for another 30 minutes in the refrigerator.

techniques for tempering

Chocolate tempering or "pre-crystallizing" can be tricky. It is necessary only for dipped or molded candy, so you don't have to worry about it if you're making most of the recipes in this book: cakes, cookies, tarts, brownies, icing, and fudge. But for bonbons, tempering creates the shine and glossy hard surface you've come to expect from great chocolate. Here's the science: Naturally fatty foods like cocoa beans or nuts separate and resist integration. The tempering process manipulates the cocoa butter molecules so that the fats and solids stay together. By putting melted chocolate through a series of temperatures (high to melt all the fats, then low to integrate and solidify the most stable fat crystals with the solids, then medium-high to create enough viscosity for handling), the chocolate stays integrated. This process is always performed at the factory, but you must perform it again if you want to reshape your chocolate, then have it set with a shiny new coat. Go with the specific temperatures given below because that's when the chemical reactions occur.

Chop. Chop 1 or 2 pounds of chocolate into very small pieces for easy melting. Place most of the chocolate in the bowl, reserving a small pile (about 1/4 of it) to cool it off later. Use a digital thermometer to test the chocolate and room temperatures throughout.

Melt. Melt the chocolate gently in a stainless steel bowl set over simmering water, or dry in a baking dish in a very low oven (ideally 115°F or the "warm" setting). Confirm the chocolate temperature reaches 115°F while stirring occasionally.

Stir, Cool, and Wait. Cool the bowl of melted chocolate by placing it in a cool spot in the kitchen (not in the refrigerator) and stirring in the remaining solid chocolate you held aside. If your room temperature is 80°F, the chocolate will eventually come down to 80°F. Ideal room temperature is about 60° to 65°F. Just stir occasionally and wait. You'll notice a slight thickening in the texture of the chocolate when it cools below 82°F. That's your cue to change directions and heat it up a little.

Heat. Heat the chocolate slightly so it becomes fluid again. The best way to do this is to put the bowl over hot water in a saucepan very briefly until it starts to warm up. You want it to be about 90°F, and stay at 90°F, so you have to "flash" the bowl on and off the hot water to keep the temperature steady. Careful, it heats up quickly!

Your chocolate is tempered, so line your molds or dip your fruit as you like. Just be aware of keeping the chocolate at 90°F—as you dip items in the chocolate, it cools.

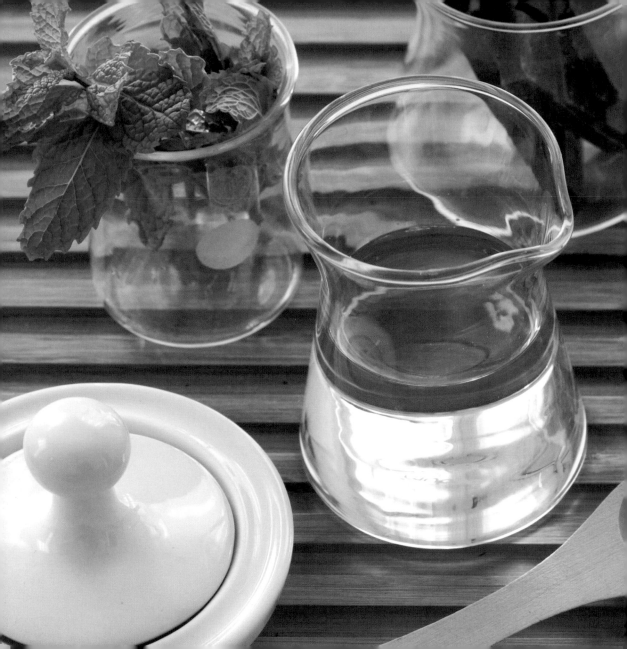

2 health and beauty

✦

HOW CHOCOLATE HELPS

YOU INSIDE AND OUT

Celebrate the chocolate gods! Their fruit is better for us than brussels sprouts! Or perhaps we should celebrate the doctors, scientists, researchers, and nutritionists who have given us study after study on the surprising health benefits of chocolate. Harvard Medical School, the Mayo Clinic, the University of California, Davis, Pennsylvania State University, and Yale Medical School, among many other institutions around the world, agree on this fact: chocolate's chemicals (specifically a class of nutrients called flavanols) contribute to our health by increasing the efficiency of blood flow to our hearts. In small dark doses, these chemicals also may be powerful antioxidant weapons in the preventive fights against cancer and aging. What's more, cocoa butter, the natural vegetable fat contained in pure chocolate, with its low melting point and rich moisture-trapping texture, has long been an effective emollient in skin care products.

how chocolate is good for you

A 1-ounce piece of very dark chocolate consumed every day provides vitamins (particularly vitamins A, D, and K), minerals (particularly magnesium, potassium, and iron), a little protein, and flavanols. Dark chocolate has more flavanols than any other type of food. Flavanols help keep blood flowing to the heart, which prevents blood clots, and they also strengthen the lining of the blood vessels. They provide antioxidant activity, which means they attract and neutralize free radicals (charged, loose electrons swimming through the bloodstream with cancer-causing potential). Further, cocoa butter has stearic and oleic acids, which are considered the "good fats," essential to a healthy body. And as we've known long before food science came along, chocolate of any kind is very good for the spirit.

Despite these healthful highlights, chocolate is not officially a health food. Cocoa beans are about half cocoa butter/fat (the rest is protein, vitamins, minerals, and carbs). That same creamy cocoa butter that softens our skin may cause us a little trouble around the waistline when we eat it, as do the delightful scoops of sugar included in most dark chocolate bars. We add more fat and sugar to chocolate when we craft it into milk chocolate or desserts. Fat and sugar are things you just won't find in brussels sprouts, and they keep chocolate off most nutritionists' lists of health foods. Despite its imperfections, chocolate, taken sensibly, is a perfectly healthful food.

But is there more? Is there a superchemical responsible for chocolate's sublime flavor and healthfulness? Is there some magic beyond the science? So far, studies have failed to yield a specific chemical, or combination, from the four hundred plus chemicals contained in chocolate, to explain its culinary appeal or health value. Carl L. Keen, chair of the Nutrition Department, University of California, Davis, conducted a comprehensive study of dietary flavanols in partnership with Mars, Inc. and Harvard Medical School in 2005. His study, along with many others, indicates that our bodies drink in enough of these powerful chemical compounds for chocolate to be considered not just healthful, but indeed medicinal. He insists the health magic of chocolate is in the flavanols. Mars, Inc. continues the quest for healthy chocolate by refining it "raw" or at temperatures low enough to preserve the maximum flavanol content in their product line, Cocoa Via. Barry Callebaut has developed a similar product, called Acticoa. Both are designed to respond to the huge demand from consumers and medical professionals for superhealthful chocolate.

How do you get the maximum benefit from eating chocolate while dodging the fatty trouble spots? You definitely need a plan.

the chocolate vitamin plan

- Think of 1 ounce of dark chocolate as a sublime vitamin you get to savor every day, you lucky creature. But it's not candy, it's a vitamin. Just take 1 dose.
- Use natural cocoa, not "Dutch-process" or "alkalized." When alkali is added to cocoa, acids are neutralized, and the cocoa turns a darker color and tastes less bitter, but many of the flavanols are also neutralized. While there are many great applications for alkalized cocoa (also known as "Dutched"), you should look for "natural" cocoa powder when you want the maximum health benefit from 1 ounce of cocoa.
- Keep a sacred stash. Store your favorite brand of dark chocolate in "daily dose" small plastic bags—exactly 1 ounce in each. Or, to be more eco-friendly, store them on seven spoons stacked together for a week's worth of chocolate vitamin intake.
- Don't substitute milk chocolate or mix chocolate with milk, cream, or butter. Candy bars and truffles don't count as chocolate vitamins since some studies show dairy products inhibit the body's ability process chocolate's most beneficial vitamins and mineral compounds. Plus they have the fat and sugar problem. Focus on dark chocolate, vitamin-style.
- Try dark chocolate with nutritious inclusions, such as nuts and dried berries. Organic brands, including Green & Black's and Dagoba, offer dark chocolate with antioxidant-rich inclusions. Plus, a snack of 1 ounce of dark chocolate with a handful of almonds, berries, or granola offers your body even more heart-friendly nutrients.
- Try a handful of cocoa nibs. These are pure pieces of cocoa bean—fermented, dried, and roasted. A 1-ounce handful will give you a crunchy, tasty dose of daily chocolate. Try finding them at your local grocery stores or go online at www.scharffenberger.com.

- Try extrahealthy chocolate formulas. Start by trying Cocoapro and CocoaVia from Mars. They are made using a process designed to retain all the healthful properties that might otherwise be processed out of chocolate. Raw or minimally roasted cacao nibs, chocolate bars, and cocoa powder are available in health food stores.
- Use chocolate as one color in your rainbow. A colorful variety of foods will assure a range of vitamin and mineral intake. Consider chocolate the dark end of your color spectrum, followed by figs, prunes, purple cabbage, beets, pomegranates, raspberries, carrots, yams, yellow squash, broccoli, kale, parsley, limes, peas, blueberries, walnuts, oatmeal, and coconut. The forces that make natural foods colorful are often the forces that make them nutritious.

Does this mean you have to give up your creamy milk chocolate bars or decadent chocolate cakes? Never! Chocolate and dairy together make sublime desserts, and the world would be a grimmer place without them. A creamy chocolate mousse has healthful properties, such as calcium from milk and protein from eggs. Chocolate itself has so many nutrients that even if some of them are inhibited by dairy products and doused with sugar, chances are you're still getting a pop of something good. But desserts are not, and never will be, health foods. The fat (lots) and sugar (tons) will get you into trouble if you don't limit them. Chocolate desserts with sugar and cream, long may they live, are on the dangerous side of chocolate's health potential. We're talking about serious limits on desserts—once a week is about all most people can afford. But that's a lot! That's 52 chocolate desserts a year, plus 365 pieces of dark chocolate. Life is good! Rich desserts are simply much better at pleasing the soul than nourishing the body.

your blood

Blood carries vitamins and minerals to all the cells of the body. It likes to flow freely, unencumbered by fat deposits or errant cells. The flavanols contained in dark chocolate work as blood thinners and cleansers. They reverse the effects of cholesterol (specifically the LDL, or low-density lipoproteins known as the bad cholesterol, which can collect and clog blood flow in the arteries). They whisk up free radicals so they will not oxidize, which is why we call flavanols "antioxidants." Flavanols also relax the walls of blood vessels, which allows more blood to flow through the arteries to the heart for maximum efficiency in the give-and-take exchange of the cardiovascular system.

your heart

Once you are in the mode of healthful living, chocolate is your best friend. By most accounts, dark chocolate has more heart-friendly nutrients than any other food, and it provides a three-way benefit for the heart: (1) flavanols keep the blood flowing smoothly in and out of the heart, also functioning with antioxidant capacity; (2) stearic acid helps counteract clumpy deposits of bad cholesterol that can pile up in the veins; and (3) chocolate creates pleasure, indeed love and joy, and nourishes the spiritual side of your heart.

Have you ever seen a human heart? It's like seeing a movie star in person—a small thing with enormous power. The curators and physicians of The Body Works, a scientific art exhibit featuring plasticized human bodies, describe it this way: "The heart is a mysterious muscle, a hard-working organ and the center of the most complex system in the human body. . . . It nourishes, regulates and sustains. . . . It is the container of our deepest emotions and highest values, the wellspring of our courage and a trusted source of deep knowledge." In the literature of our arts and sciences, the heart bypasses the brain as a symbol of the emotional essence of a person.

But what about *your* heart? Since coronary heart disease is the number-one killer of Americans and Europeans, doctors warn about the dangers of neglected hearts. If you do not exercise your heart—awaken it fully every day with rushes of blood from vigorous activities—your heart will lose its power. It needs to be toned and conditioned, yet like all of our muscles, it is quite happy to relax and do nothing. So you have to keep it strong. You might as well participate in a heart-healthy lifestyle or you can't really use dark chocolate and red wine for the medicinal value they offer.

Joyfulness is also important to your heart. Studies on the health properties of red wine often note the context of typical wine drinking: in a relaxed environment, after work and stress, with friends and family, with great food. We connect with loved ones over food, we cook together, we relax when we're with friends in a restaurant. Even eating alone can bring a pure pleasure in food that feeds the engine of happiness. Indulging in a decadent dessert can be a shared splurge with friends

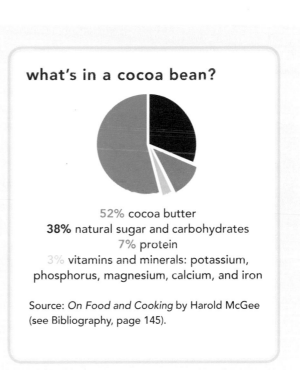

what's in a cocoa bean?

52% cocoa butter
38% natural sugar and carbohydrates
7% protein
3% vitamins and minerals: potassium, phosphorus, magnesium, calcium, and iron

Source: *On Food and Cooking* by Harold McGee (see Bibliography, page 145).

or a spiritual indulgence in your self-worth. Celebration and moderate indulgence in satisfying foods are indeed good for all aspects of your heart, and this includes chocolate desserts.

your skin

Skin is your biggest, heaviest organ. It is the warm blanket that holds all your pulsing parts together. Two options exist for long-term skin care: embrace medical technology (chemical peels, laser resurfacing, collagen injections, botox, and surgical facelifts) or embrace natural nurturing (as many aromatic facials and massages as you can possibly afford). Skin care products made with chocolate can smooth your skin, impart nutrients, and awaken your senses. But can they make your skin look younger? Feel younger? Erase laugh lines or unfurrow a thoughtful brow? I asked my dermatologist if the best of balms, lotions, creams, or serums could manage my wrinkling issues, and he just laughed. The natural/nuturing approach involves a big embrace of inner beauty! Yet of the two options, it has much to recommend it.

Surgery, unfortunately, fails at providing the luster we seek for our skin, what Shakespeare simply calls the "rose of youth." Explorers sought the fountain of youth well before Shakespeare's time, and not even the vitamin-packed cacao bean and other exotic treasures they stumbled upon can prevent our skin and bodies from aging. So let's accept that neither natural beauty treatments nor plastic surgery will eliminate aging, although studies suggest antioxidant-rich diets can help slow it. Mostly, natural products will mitigate it, soften it, scent it, and allow us to accept age in our faces as we accept it deeply in ourselves. This is the essence of the spa experience.

The Global Spa Economy Report announced that in 2007 spas worldwide generated $60.3 billion in core industry revenues, from facilities, capital investments, education, consulting, media, associations, and events. Spa-related hospitality, tourism, and real estate generated another whopping $194 billion. The wellness business is a modern bonanza, but its philosophies are grounded in old ways. Ancient Greek, Roman, and early civilizations of Asia embraced the practice of relaxing, rejuvenating, and maintaining health through

peacefulness, aromatic baths, mindful eating, and pleasing activities. They indulged the senses with calmness and beauty as a technique for good living. Today, the tending of body, soul, skin, and spirit are part of a thriving luxury industry that embraces another thriving luxury industry: chocolate.

Healing properties of chocolate skin care relate to the theory of medicating the body externally. Our seven layers of skin are very porous and absorb many things we put on them. Think of how many medicines are applied through a skin patch—nicotine for smokers, pain-relieving chemicals for cancer patients. Yet are enough of chocolate's vitamins absorbed through the skin to make a difference? Do antioxidants need to be processed through the cardiovascular system to generate benefits? Research on the skin's ability to absorb antioxidants in dosages high enough to penetrate the cardiovascular system is still underway, and the results, like so many regarding chocolate and health, are inconclusive. We know chocolate's antioxidant power theoretically can slow the aging process, so the race is on to get measurable results. In the meantime, we can take comfort in cocoa butter's proven ability to soothe the outer layers of our skin. Facial creams, moisturizers, and lotions made with natural cocoa butter melt easily on the skin, hold moisture, protect us from harsh elements, feel rich and smooth, and offer the pleasing aroma of chocolate.

Nerve endings just under the skin send messages of pain, pleasure, and peace directly to the brain. The skin itself is sensitive and lets you know pretty quickly if it is irritated. So if a product feels good, smells good, soothes your skin, and pleases your senses, it is good for you. For a list of spa practitioners who will massage you with chocolate-scented oil or wrap you in chocolate fondue, simply check an online search engine for "chocolate facial + [city]", and you will find a chocolate-enlightened spa near you or your travel destination.

ultimate in-home chocolate spa

You can lift your spirits by transforming your bathroom into a decadent den of cocoa. In my personal journey through pools of chocolate baths and beauty products, these are my very favorites:

Chocolate candles from Chocolate Flower Farm at www.chocolateflowerfarm.com.

Chocolate Mousse Hydration Masque by Éminence Organic Skin Care at www.eminenceorganics.com.

Chocolate Soap (see recipe, page 70).

Cocoa Butter Moisturizing Soap in a Tin from Asquith and Somerset, available at www.shoplondons.com/cocoa.html.

Hint of Cocoa Body Lotion (see recipe, page 65).

Hot Chocolate Sugar Scrub from Giovanni Cosmetics at www.giovannicosmetics.com.

Lip balm from Scharffen Berger at www.scharffenberger.com.

Melt Away Chocolate Massage Oil (see recipe, page 66).

Queen Helene Cocoa Butter Body Lotion at www.queenhelene.com/naturals.

your teeth

Back in the Dark Ages, before healthful chocolate became part of our lexicon, it was lumped in with delightful, tooth-destroying sugary foods like Starburst Fruit Chews, SweeTarts, and Sugar Babies. But in the flurry of research conducted on chocolate in the last decade, a surprising fact emerged: Chocolate, by itself, is not bad for your teeth because the high quantity of cocoa butter prevents it from sticking to your teeth at all. So it's a sweet, sugary product that washes away before the sugar particles can attach themselves to the teeth, burrow in, and cause the plaque that dental hygienists complain about when you are imprisoned in the dental chair. Researchers in Japan also found that the husks of cocoa beans—usually thrown away in production—help the mouth fight plaque-causing bacteria and have potential as an active ingredient in mouthwash. While no studies go as far as to claim chocolate's benefits for oral health offset the dangers of sugar, at least you can accept that chocolate is not the biggest tooth decay culprit.

your brain

Some of chocolate's chemical compounds are psychoactive, which means, in the right doses, they can alter the way you think, feel, and perceive the world. You may have heard the rumors about the natural high triggered by chocolate's chemicals. Especially on the Internet, chocolate is often referred to as a "mood food" containing the "love drug." Fortunately, your brain has one very effective tool: common sense. When you see a headline announcing that chocolate makes you high, you'll remember the last time you enjoyed a chocolate bar and say to yourself, "It tasted good. It made me happy. It satisfied me. But high? Probably not."

Chocolate does indeed have powerful chemicals: tryptophan, anandamide, caffeine, endorphins, and phenylethylamines. Tryptophan, like marijuana, triggers the neurotransmitter serotonin—except you would have to eat about 5 pounds of chocolate in one sitting to get a psychoactive effect or a high. Anandamide is a marijuana-like chemical, also in small quantities; caffeine is the same stimulating alkaloid found in your morning cup of coffee, only less; endorphins are a family of peptides released by the brain that act as opiates; and phenylethylamine is the "love drug" related to the release of brain dopamine experienced by people falling in love. Yet cheddar cheese and salami contain more phenylethylamine than chocolate, and the idea of a cheddar- and salami-flavored love haze is not quite as sexy as the chocolate-inspired theory. So while we are all intrigued by the discovery of mood-altering chemicals in chocolate, current science insists that it is not making us high, addicted, lovesick, or even a little tipsy.

> The setting sun, and music at the close
> As the last taste of sweets, is sweetest last,
> Writ in remembrance more than things long past.
>
> —William Shakespeare, *Richard II*

Studies find that brain stimulation comes from the pleasure of eating chocolate—the aroma, the flavors, the mouthfeel, the memories—not the actual traces of psychoactive chemicals. In other words, the sensuous pleasures, not the chemicals, make us love chocolate. David Benton, professor of psychology at the University College of Wales, in conjunction with the International Cocoa Manufacturers Association, analyzed all the data available on chocolate, its chemicals, cravings, and addictions and concluded, "All palatable foods stimulate endorphin release in the brain and this is the most likely mechanism to account for the elevation of mood. . . . For many, chocolate offers a near optimally pleasant taste that potently stimulates endorphin release in the brain. There is no convincing evidence that there are substances in chocolate that act directly on the brain in a pharmacological manner."

what to believe?

Now, some tricky questions relevant to all scientific studies: Who paid for the research? Who stands to profit from results indicating that chocolate is healthful or psychoactive? What methods were used in the surveys, tests, and studies? Must we accept all this news about chocolate's health benefits without a grain of salt? Chocolate companies themselves provide most of the funding for research. This, as critics point out, can lead to biased results. When food trends moved away from sugar and fat, chocolate sales stalled. But with the advent of health news about flavanols and antioxidants, sales, particularly of premium dark chocolate, shot up. This echoes the boost of red wine sales once its health benefits were established. Giant global chocolate corporations enjoy this health news and the subsequent profits, and they want more of both. If chocolate becomes an established natural pharmaceutical, not just a snack, two new lines of business open up for them: chocolate health food and chocolate medicine. The chocolate companies are, therefore, motivated. Yet underneath all this cynicism and profit drive is also goodwill, which is why the medical institutions have a big stake, too. If the chemicals in chocolate can be further manipulated to fight heart disease, cancer, immune system disorders, or depression, the citizens of the world will benefit. The investments of these chocolate companies and many major medical and scientific

> **bliss byte: chef's quote**
>
> Chocolate is a complex ingredient. It's tricky. I find it both energizing and calming.
>
> —Chef Josh Needleman, Chocolate Springs, Lenox, Massachusetts

institutions help harness chocolate's health powers. Most studies in the field cite the need for further research, so the process is in its early stages. As much as we have to be cautious about every health claim we see in the papers, the chocolate companies, as they explore business opportunities, are doing a lot of good work.

controlling cravings

Don't even bother trying to separate food and feelings. They are together from birth. Our first food, mother's milk, is sweet. Anthropologists believe that since good food sources for early man, like berries and nontoxic plants, were also sweet, we evolved to connect sweetness with survival. Sugar also indicates foods with nutrients: fruits, vegetables, grains, milk. As for our relationship with chocolate, it, too, begins early in life—you know it as the beloved chips in your cookies, a welcome warm drink after school or a day of skiing in winter, a Halloween delight, or maybe a little treat from your mom. So as you walk around craving a candy bar, your instincts are leading you to something both nutritional and emotional.

Close to 96 percent of the population experiences food cravings, and chocolate tops the list of all foods craved by far. Despite years of research, scientists have not found the single component that causes this, nor have they found that chocolate cravings stem from nutritional deficiencies that would cause the body to self-medicate. What we know about chocolate and cravings, much of it from data in the fields of clinical health, psychological health, nutrition, and ongoing biological research, dovetails with what we know about chocolate and brain chemicals. It is the complete package of chocolate eating—the pleasure of the flavor, the psychological associations, those satisfying fats, the perfect sweetness, and the battalion of nutrients—that lock into a unit of effectiveness. Take away any one of those components, and you

make peace with friendly fats

Some fattening foods, including dark chocolate, avocados, almonds, walnuts, olives, and olive oil, are so full of nutrients that you should eat them anyway. You can't eat tons of them—just small amounts. These foods contain monosaturated fats (also know as "the good fat"). Another type of fat is saturated fat (also known as "the bad fat"). Transfats can now be considered "the worst fat" because they are chemically engineered for shelf life and low cost and are practically indigestible for the body. Cocoa butter is a good vegetable fat even though some of its elements fall in the saturated fat category. It's still a fat. If you eat too much of it, it will make you, well, fat. But in moderation, the fat from chocolate's cocoa butter, especially in dark chocolate, is healthful.

won't have as much kick. We crave chocolate because it is a complex, powerfully integrated, uniquely pleasing food.

Myths of chocolate cravings and women abound: women crave chocolate more than men; women crave chocolate before their periods; chocolate reduces anxiety; chocolate cravings are caused by hormones. While women crave chocolate more than men, the guys are in the game. About 97 percent of women have food cravings, as do 68 percent of men. Chocolate is the most craved food by both genders, with cookies, cakes, and chips rounding out the winner's circle.

Now that we've established that chocolate cravings are a fact of life for most of us, how should we manage them? Nutrition experts advise to give in—eat a small portion of the food you crave—which relieves the tendencies toward binging, denial, and obsession. For chocolate lovers, this synchronizes with scientific advice to eat small servings of dark chocolate daily to maximize health benefits for the heart and bloodstream. Managing your chocolate desires can lead you to managing your health. You can indulge in the pleasures of chocolate—albeit by a very specific set of indulgence rules—and you can accept that chocolate is a healthful part of your life. News from nutritionists doesn't get much better than this.

K. Dun Gifford, founder of Oldways Preservation Trust, a think tank devoted to healthful food advocacy, believes in allowing the pleasure of food to be part of a nutritious eating regime. He suggests, "We must manage our sugar like we manage other things in life: anger, checkbooks, calories, marriage, speed, relationships, sun exposure, homework, work assignments, and alcohol." He supports a Mediterranean-style diet rich in olive oil, fish, vegetables, and legumes. Desserts, and all the joy they symbolize, are part of this vision.

Michael Schneider, publisher of *Dessert Professional* magazine, agrees. As he watches the food trends spark around chocolate and sugar, he resists scientific assessments. He likes the French model in which people make simple desserts with very high-quality ingredients and enjoy them profoundly. "Chocolate has a natural beauty and puts a smile on your face. If you're on a diet, get a great dessert and just eat half."

With all things chocolate, common sense must prevail. A little chocolate in the body and on the skin is good for you, but you still have to eat a lot of other nutritious food like broccoli, drink a lot of water, do your cardio, floss your teeth, and pay your bills. Great chocolate is a part of a good-living health plan.

healthy recipes: from snacks to skin care

These recipes celebrate the healthful properties of chocolate. The first group pairs chocolate with other foods high in antioxidants. The second group incorporates chocolate and/or cocoa butter into handmade bath and beauty products designed to bring the goodness of chocolate to the heart through the skin.

chocolate balsamic vinaigrette

What better way to indulge in a little chocolate than by adding it to a plethora of healthy greens, pine nuts, and feta cheese? You'll be looking for an excuse to eat your vegetables with this surprising twist on vinaigrette. **Makes 1 cup salad dressing; serves large salad for 10**

Put all the ingredients into a blender and blend on low until mixed, less than a minute.

2 tablespoons balsamic vinegar

2 tablespoons rice wine vinegar (or white vinegar)

1 ounce dark chocolate, melted

2 tablespoons water

1/2 cup extra virgin olive oil

1 teaspoon minced garlic

1 teaspoon kosher salt

Ground pepper to taste

blueberry cocoa nib crumble

It was summer in New England the first time I read about the health benefits of blueberries. I rushed to the pick-your-own patch on a nearby hill. I put several perfect ones in my palm with all their little hats aligned—an army of antioxidant soldiers. I ate them. Sweet, with a tang. Yet, sadly, I felt nothing. My blood did not quicken; my heart did not swell with strength. I was my just my same old self, munching a handful of blueberries by the side of the road. In my chocolate research, this moment comes to mind often. The benefits of chocolate arrive quietly amid a myriad of other healthful living components. Health through chocolate is a practice. Chocolate and blueberries, both miracles of nature, join here for a berry breakfast or homey, warm dessert. **Makes 8 servings**

Blueberry Base

2 pints fresh blueberries

2 tablespoons sugar

2 tablespoons whole wheat flour

1 tablespoon vanilla extract

1 teaspoon ground cinnamon

1/2 teaspoon kosher salt

Zest from 1/2 lemon, finely grated

Juice from 1/2 lemon

Crumble

3/4 cup rolled oats, chopped

1/2 cup whole wheat flour

1/4 cup firmly packed light brown sugar

1/2 cup confectioners' sugar

1 teaspoon ground cinnamon

1/2 teaspoon baking powder

1/2 cup cocoa nibs

3/4 cup crushed pecans

1/2 teaspoon kosher salt

1/2 cup (1 stick) cold unsalted butter, chopped into small pieces

Whipped cream or vanilla bean ice cream, to serve

Preheat the oven to 350°F.

To prepare the blueberries, in a medium bowl, toss together the blueberries, sugar, flour, vanilla, cinnamon, salt, zest, and lemon juice. Transfer the mixture to an 8 or 9-inch pie plate or small baking dish and set aside. Rinse out the bowl to use for the crumble, keeping kitchen mess to a minimum.

For the crumble, mix together the oats, flour, brown sugar, confectioners' sugar, cinnamon, baking powder, cocoa nibs, pecans, salt, and butter in the bowl.

Toss them together like you would a salad. Then pour the mixture over the blueberry base.

Bake for 1 hour. Serve hot and bubbly. It goes especially well with vanilla bean ice cream. If you want a more formal presentation, allow the dessert to cool to room temperature and decorate it with piped whipped cream and fresh blueberries.

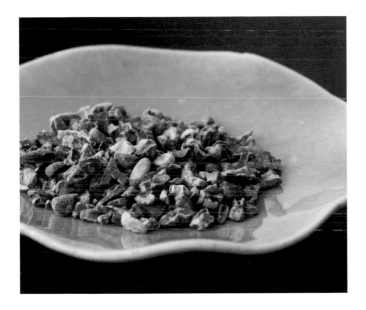

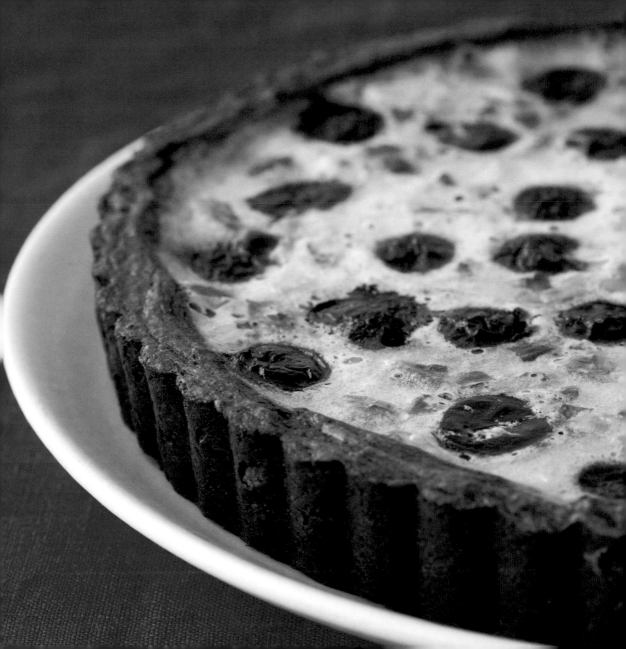

cherry tart with cocoa nib crust

Chocolate crust cradles a bevy of "superfoods," including almonds, cherries, and eggs. Inspired by the French classic *clafoutis*, this tart is "choc full" of cherries. They float jewel-like inside a sweet, vanilla-scented custard. By the way, here are three good ways to pit a cherry: (1) Use an old-fashioned vegetable peeler that has a curved edge on top to scratch around the top of the cherry pit, then dig around the stone, scoop under it, and it will pop right out; (2) use a paring knife as above (but watch out—it's easy to slice your fingertips); (3) use a cherry-pitter carried by some gourmet kitchen stores—a special tool invented just for this job! This recipe requires only half a batch of the Chocolate Sugar Dough—make a full batch and freeze half for future crust or cookie needs.

Makes 1 (9-inch) tart

To prepare the crust, make the Chocolate Sugar Dough. Knead in the cocoa nibs. Press the dough into a flat disk, wrap with plastic or place in a sealable plastic freezer bag, and chill for 20 minutes or so. Roll out the dough on a lightly floured piece of parchment paper or flat surface to about 1/2 inch thick. Transfer to a tart pan (9 inches in diameter, 2 inches deep) by loosening the dough from the work surface with an offset spatula, then sliding the tart pan under it. Once you smooth the dough in the tart pan (pinching any rips or cracks together with your fingers), line the top of the dough with a layer of almonds, lightly pressing them into the dough. Cover this prepared tart shell with plastic wrap and put in the refrigerator.

Preheat the oven to 300°F.

To make the custard, combine the milk and cream in a small saucepan with the vanilla bean pod and seeds. Bring the mixture to a simmer.

continued

Crust
1 pound Chocolate Sugar Dough (page 132)

1/2 cup cocoa nibs

1/2 cup chopped almonds

Custard
1/2 cup milk

1/2 cup heavy cream

1 vanilla bean, split and seeded

3 large eggs

3 tablespoons sugar

3 tablespoons arrowroot or cornstarch

1/2 teaspoon almond extract

1 teaspoon nut liqueur (such as Frangelico or Amaretto) (optional)

1 teaspoon kosher salt

2 cups pitted sour cherries (preferably fresh, or frozen)

Meanwhile, briskly whisk together the eggs, sugar, arrowroot, almond extract, nut liqueur, and salt in a bowl. Remove the vanilla bean pod from the hot milk mixture and slowly pour one-third of the hot milk mixture into the egg mixture and continue to whisk. Repeat this process two more times and stir until the batter is smooth.

Remove the prepared tart shell from the refrigerator and remove the plastic wrap. Put the cherries in the shell. Then pour the batter over the cherries and allow the mixture to rest for about a minute. Place a cake pan half full of water in the oven to keep the oven moist. Place the tart pan in the oven and bake for about 40 minutes, or until the custard is lightly browned and solid, with no liquid jiggle in the center.

Allow the tart to cool in the pan to room temperature before serving.

bliss byte: chef's quote

We must be patient with the chocolate.

—Chef Laurent Pages, Barry Callebaut Chocolate Academy, Canada

craving kicker cocoa cookies

You'll get a crunchy cocoa kick and a buttery, sweet finish from these iced chocolate sugar cookies. They're small enough that if you eat one or two, you'll have satisfaction, not guilt. Make a full batch of dough and freeze half for later use. **Makes 25 to 30 cookies**

Make the Chocolate Sugar Dough and allow it to chill for at least 30 minutes as directed.

Preheat the oven to 350°F. Line two cookie sheets with parchment paper or silicone baking mats.

Put the dough on a floured piece of parchment paper or a silicone baking mat. Dust a little flour on top of the cold dough, cover with another piece of parchment paper or silicone mat, and roll the dough with a rolling pin until it is about 1/4 inch thick. Use a cookie cutter to cut the shapes and place them on the prepared cookie sheet about 1/2 inch apart. If the dough gets too soft and sticky as you work, chill it for 20 minutes and try again.

Bake the cookies for about 10 minutes, or until they are set. Prepare the icing as you allow them to cool on the baking sheet. Once they are close to room temperature and sturdy, transfer them to a plate from which you can easily pick them up and ice them. Repeat this process until all your dough has been rolled out and baked.

Prepare the icing as directed and flavor it with something to elevate your mood— maybe coffee, maybe whiskey, maybe honey. Maybe a bit of all three! The icing is very versatile so you can adjust it to suit your taste. When the cookies are cool, spread a thin layer on each one with a small offset spatula or dinner knife. Then dust them with a touch of cocoa powder or sandwich them together for a double dose of the chocolate cure. Unused icing freezes well.

Chocolate Choices

Valrhona cocoa powder for the dough; Endangered Species milk chocolate and Trader Joe's 72% dark chocolate for the icing

1 pound Chocolate Sugar Dough (page 132)

3 cups Simple Secret Icing (page 136)

1 tablespoon strong brewed coffee (optional)

1 tablespoon whiskey (optional)

1 tablespoon honey (optional)

Cocoa powder, to dust (optional)

dangerous date dots

These easy, no-bake candies are good for you if you eat only two or three, which is dangerously difficult to do. You'll find a balance between the natural sweetness of dates and honey and the bitterness of rich cocoa. **Makes 24 (1/2-inch) pieces**

1/2 cup almonds

1/2 cup roasted, salted cashews

10 dates (preferably Medjool), pitted

3 tablespoons agave syrup or honey

1 teaspoon vanilla extract

2 tablespoons unsweetened cocoa powder

1/2 cup shredded coconut

2 tablespoons cocoa butter (or a flavorless oil, such as canola or safflower)

Toasted ribbon, flaked, or sliced coconut, for garnish

Combine the almonds and cashews in a food processor and pulse until finely chopped. Add the dates, agave syrup, vanilla, cocoa powder, and 1/4 cup of the shredded coconut and pulse until combined. Melt the cocoa butter, pour into the mixture, and process until smooth. Form into the shape of a log about 1 inch in diameter, wrap in plastic, and chill for about 20 minutes.

Unwrap the log and slice it into even 1/2-inch pieces. Take each piece and roll it between your palms until it forms a compact ball. Decorate each ball with the remaining 1/4 cup shredded coconut and the ribbon coconut.

diet day dip

Some days, the fats and sugars of life must be avoided, but you can still squeeze in a little chocolate. I usually prefer natural ingredients like whole milk and real sugar, but on diet day, everything must be skinny, and I use sugar substitutes. Swirl a green apple slice through this dip in the afternoon, make a cup of green tea, soak up all your antioxidants, and you'll forget that you're even on a diet. **Makes 1/2 cup dip**

Sift the cocoa powder in a small bowl and slowly pour the hot milk over it. Whisk together until smooth. Whisk in the yogurt, sweetener, vanilla, and salt. Serve with fruit slices.

Chocolate Choices

Scharffen Berger or Hershey's unsweetened cocoa powder; should be a "natural" or "nonalkalized" cocoa powder

1/4 cup unsweetened cocoa powder

1/4 cup skim milk, hot

3 tablespoons low-fat vanilla yogurt

11/2 tablespoons diet sweetener, such as Equal or Splenda

1/2 teaspoon vanilla extract

1/4 teaspoon kosher salt

Sliced fruit, to serve

sugarplum sauce

Sugarplums, made famous by the "Dance of the Sugarplum Fairy" in Tchaikovsky's ballet, *The Nutcracker Suite*, is an old-fashioned English word for candy. It evokes the sweet glory of a dried plum, also known as a prune. Lately, body-cleansing properties of prunes have made them embarrassing. But so what if they are healthy? They are also beautifully sweet like candy, full of wrinkle-fighting antioxidants, and charged with fiber and vitamins. In this recipe, with an assist from dark chocolate, prunes regain their rightful place as sugarplums. This sauce makes a fine duet with ice cream or a slice of pound cake (see Breakfast-in-Bed Pound Cake, page 26). **Makes 1 cup sauce**

Chocolate Choices

Ghirardelli Premium, E. Guittard, Omahene, or Green & Black's dark chocolate

10 prunes, thinly sliced lengthwise

3 tablespoons maple syrup

3 tablespoons water

1/4 cup brewed coffee

3 tablespoon light brown sugar

1 tablespoon Cognac

3 ounces dark chocolate, finely chopped

Combine the prunes, maple syrup, water, coffee, and brown sugar in a small saucepan and bring to a boil. Boil for about 3 minutes, lower the heat, and add the Cognac and dark chocolate. Stir until you have a smooth consistency. Serve warm over ice cream or cake.

Chocolate's aromas will fill your kitchen as you prepare these products, then scent your bathroom with cocoa every time you use them. And they make great gifts!

hint of cocoa body lotion

Good news for dry-skinned chocolate aficionados! Cocoa butter is one of the best fats you can use to hydrate the body, plus you get a faint, natural scent of cocoa. (But no tasting—it's got chemicals to preserve it!) This lotion, an emulsion between fat and liquid, is suitable for everyday use. Pump-top bottles are available in beauty supply stores and some pharmacies. For cocoa butter and chocolate extract sources, see Shopping Sources Guide, page 142. **Makes 1 1/4 cups lotion**

Melt the cocoa butter in the microwave on low heat for 1 minute in an ovenproof measuring cup or other micro-wavable container. Stir, then use 30-second blasts as needed until the cocoa butter is a smooth yellow liquid. Stir in the grapeseed oil. Transfer to a blender and allow the mixture to cool for several minutes.

Meanwhile, combine the water and borax in a small saucepan and bring to a boil over medium heat. Run the blender at medium speed for a few seconds, then stop it and add a splash of the boiling water, then run it again for several seconds. This is a gradual way to create the emulsion between fat and water, and the borax helps holds them together. Once all the water is added, continue blending, adding the chocolate extract and the vanilla extract. The mixture should look white and frothy. Transfer the lotion to a pump-top bottle. It thickens up a bit as it cools. Shake it again before using to refresh the emulsion.

1/2 cup cocoa butter

1/2 cup grapeseed oil

2/3 cup water

1/2 teaspoon borax (a salt-like chemical available in the cleansers section of supermarkets)

1 tablespoon chocolate extract

1 teaspoon vanilla extract

chocolate mint foot rub

Start with a simple, odorless lotion, or use a foot lotion that already contains strong peppermint extracts, such as the Body Shop's Peppermint Cooling Foot Lotion (see Shopping Sources Guide, page 143). Or, why not make your own lotion? See page 65 for Hint of Cocoa Body Lotion. **Makes 1 cup foot rub**

1 cup odorless or mint lotion

3 drops peppermint extract

1 1/2 ounces dark chocolate, melted

Pour the contents of a small bottle of lotion (about 1 cup) into a small bowl. Add the peppermint extract and the chocolate, then stir together. Return the lotion to the bottle using a pastry bag or a sealable plastic bag with the corner snipped out.

melt away chocolate massage oil

When you make your own massage oil, you'll experience surprising warmth, richness, and childlike feelings of happiness—similar to the well-being that a cup of hot cocoa brings. Antioxidant rich, all-natural grapeseed and almond oils help transport your body and soul to a place of sweet relaxation. This massage oil is very dark brown and brings a light brown color to your skin that easily can transfer to towels or clothes—after all, you are slathered in chocolate! Rinse off with warm wet cloths or a hot shower before you face the world. **Makes 2 1/2 cups massage oil**

2 tablespoons unsweetened cocoa powder

2 1/2 ounces dark chocolate, melted

1 cup grapeseed oil

1 cup sweet almond oil

1 teaspoon vanilla extract

In a small bowl, mix the cocoa powder into the chocolate. Slowly pour in the grapeseed oil, then the sweet almond oil, then the vanilla extract. Once the mixture is combined, you can transfer it to a plastic squeeze bottle for easy application as massage oil, or put it in a jar, label it, and offer it as a gift to a massage-needy person.

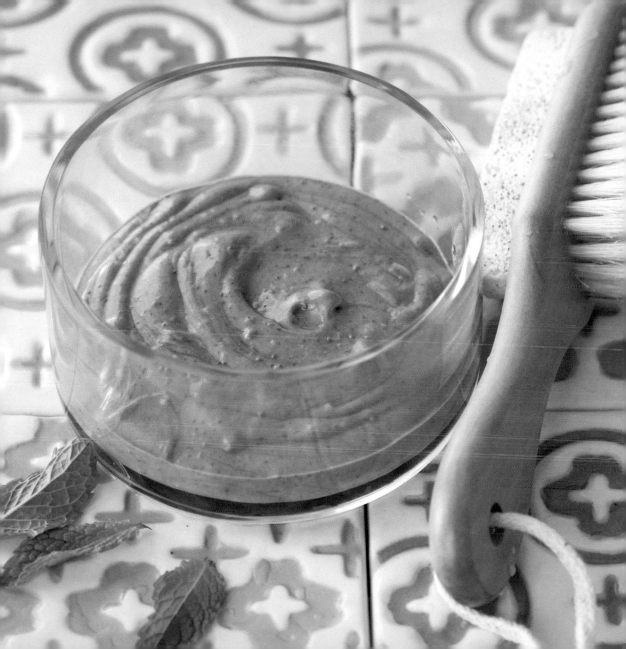

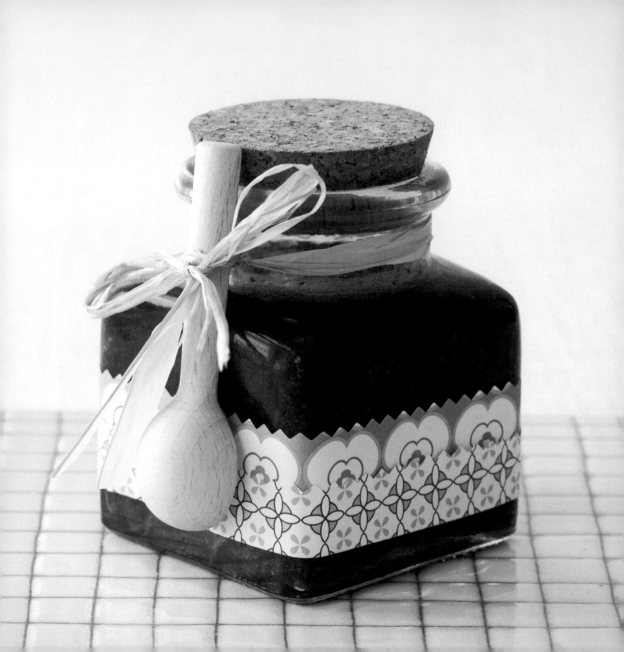

salty chocolate body scrub

You'll get some scratchy texture from this exfoliating salt scrub, which should be followed by a warm rinse for a lingering, silky texture on the skin. You'll find the oils for this recipe in health food stores. The treatment works best at the end of a hot bath. For a less expensive version, use either almond or jojoba oil (instead of both). **Makes 2 1/2 cups scrub**

Use a food processor or blender to grind the oats into a powder. Add the cocoa nibs, cocoa powder, salt, almond oil, jojoba oil, and vitamin E oil. Hit pulse a few times to blend.

Store in a glass or plastic jar, and scoop out for use with a spoon or a seashell. Massage the scrub into skin, then rinse with warm water.

1/2 cup rolled oats

1/2 cup cocoa nibs

2 tablespoons unsweetened cocoa powder

1/2 cup kosher salt

1/2 cup sweet almond oil

1/2 cup jojoba oil

2 tablespoons vitamin E oil

chocolate soap

Bring the goodness of chocolate to your own soap with this simple recipe. You'll be tempted to wash your mouth out with this soap . . . but don't! **Makes 1 1/2 pounds soap**

16 ounces unscented soap base, such as shea butter soap (see Shopping Sources Guide, page 143)

6 ounces dark chocolate, melted

2 tablespoons chocolate extract

Seeds of 1 vanilla bean

Put the soap base in a big microwave-safe measuring cup or bowl. Melt according to the instructions on the package, or until it is liquid. Stir in the chocolate, chocolate extract, and vanilla bean seeds. Mix until all the ingredients are combined. Pour the mixture into soap molds or a 9-inch cake pan, and allow the chocolate soap to set at room temperature for about 1/2 hour. Then break up the soap and wrap it in individual pieces or cut out shapes with a cookie cutter.

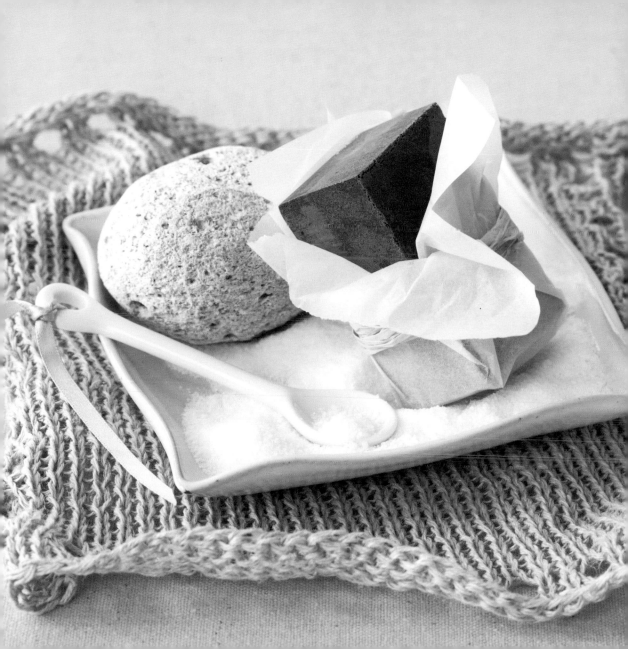

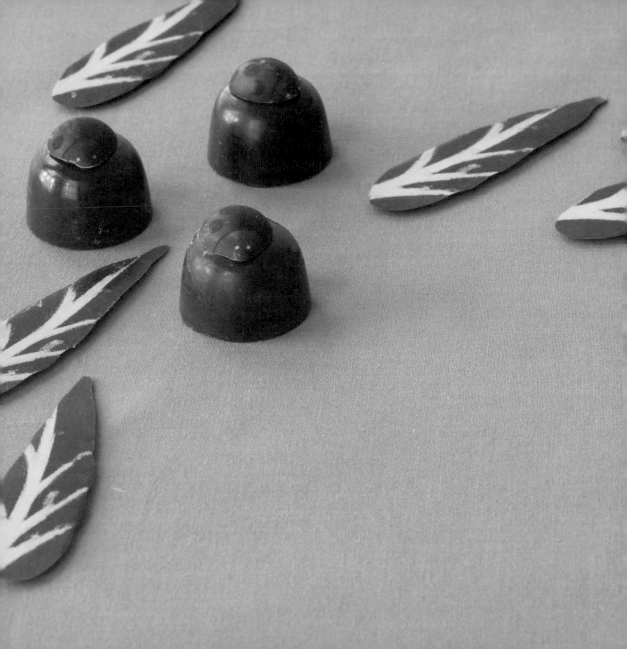

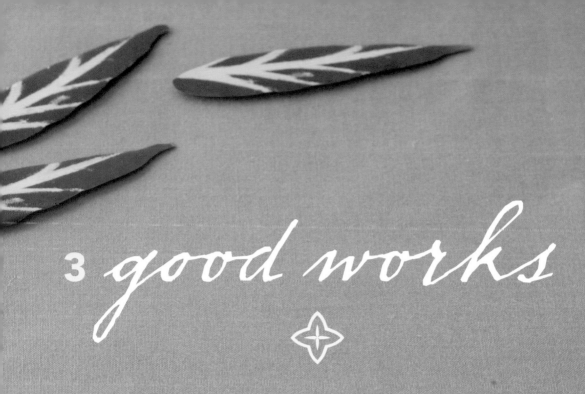

3 *good works*

✦

HOW YOU CAN HELP CHOCOLATE

Your chocolate begins in the jungles of Africa or Indonesia or South America, where most people live in grinding poverty. The cocoa beans travel from the jungle down a washed-out dirt road on the back of a truck, through villages with no schools or potable water. Much of the surrounding terrain is stripped forest, supporting cattle farms or timber operations. The original rain forests, which sustained cacao production for centuries, are in danger of being forever lost to the world.

The ongoing population explosion means more people need more timber, more sugar cane, more rubber for tires, and more cattle for fast food burgers than ever before. The rain forest jungles, sources for these needed products, at one time seemed limitless. Slash and burn techniques (burning huge plots of land then converting them to farms) and monocropping (clearing, then installing single-crop plantations) developed as efficient means to employ land quickly and meet the world's demands. These quick-clearing techniques provided landowners or rogue raiders very fast profits in very poor regions of Brazil and the Amazon jungles of Venezuela. But if you slash or burn down all the trees and develop the land for cattle grazing or single crops, the delicate nutrient system that spawned the original forest is damaged and the forest will not return until all the cattle and crops move on, and perhaps not at all. If and when it does return, it is degraded and may never be able to support its original diversity of flora and fauna. In short, these techniques are not sustainable.

The Food and Agricultural Organization of the United Nations estimates that approximately 26 million acres of tropical forest were permanently destroyed each year in the period from 2000 to 2005, most of them in chocolate's growing regions. Trees are one of the few resources we have to address global warming, and thus this level of deforestation is considered a crisis. The appetite for undeveloped land of rain forests is still growing, just as the world needs the forest intact more than ever.

Chocolate is part of the solution. Because cacao trees grow best when all of the elements of the rain forest are together, they preserve the delicate rain forest ecosystem. Further, cacao is a cash crop that can provide long-term profits for farmers. Cacao trees bear fruit for decades, while the profits for logging and cattle farming are steep but short-term because of land depletion. Educating farmers, potential farmers, and landowners of these realities is part of the promise of chocolate.

vanilla: chocolate's jungle sidekick

Mesoamericans developed both cacao and vanilla, which grew wild in southern Mexico. They were used together in *chocoatl*, the famous chocolate drink of those ancient cultures. The Spanish conquistadores named vanilla after the scabbards of their swords, or "little scabbard." People believed in its powers as an aphrodisiac, so its name and symbolism are all the more intriguing.

Once these twin delicacies—chocolate and vanilla—met the hands of French pastry chefs in imperial Europe in the 1700s, another phase of their relationship began. Auguste Escoffier, founding hero of haute cuisine, later featured several chocolate desserts in his famous cookbook *Le Guide Culinaire*—and where there is chocolate, there is always vanilla.

The painstaking work of vanilla harvesting and curing is akin to the work of turning cacao into chocolate. Because of the careful hand-pollination necessary to make the timid flowers bear fruit, vanilla is one of the most expensive spices in the world. Like cacao, vanilla thrives in diverse rain forest environments. Today vanilla grows primarily in Mexico, Indonesia, Tahiti, Réunion, and Madagascar.

How to Split and Seed Vanilla Beans. To get the seeds out, place the vanilla bean pod on a cutting board and hold it with one thumb. Puncture the top of the pod near your thumb and slice it all the way down. Then pry the pod open with both hands. Next, place your thumb in the same spot with the open pod (split side up) on the cutting board. With your other hand, hold the paring knife with the back of the blade pressed down on the inside of the pod and scrape all the way down. The black little dots that collect on your knife blade are your precious vanilla beans.

the trees

Cacao trees have a lot of attitude—they only grow in a band of tropical countries 20 degrees north or south of the equator (specifically Brazil, Cameroon, Costa Rica, Ecuador, Ghana, Ivory Coast, Madagascar, Malaysia, Mexico, Nigeria, Indonesia, and Venezuela, plus a few others). They refuse to bear fruit anywhere else. They like other trees around to protect them from wind, and they are susceptible to devastating fungal infestations, such as witches broom and black pod, against which they have no defense. They are part of an extremely diverse rain forest ecosystem with three main layers in humid, rainy climates. The top layer is a canopy of hard woods and big trees called "mother trees" because they provide shade and nourishment for the layers below. Chocolate lives in the next layer down along with bananas, ferns, palms, and orchids. The third and lowest forest floor layer is deep with leaves, mulch, rotting fruit, sticks, and bugs such as the midge, a tiny gnatlike insect that pollinates cacao's flowers and turns them into fruit-bearing pods. This bottom layer is also an essential fertilizer for cacao growth. So if you want to eat chocolate—and don't we all—you have to support all the bugs and trees and mulch and wildlife around the trees that make the harvest possible. You and your chocolate are locked together in a strategic green future.

"Chocolate can change the world for the better," says Alexander Morozoff, executive editor and publisher of *Cocoaroma*, the photographic travel guide to fine choco-

> ## bliss byte: chef's quote
>
> I have always had a love affair with chocolate, and my Honduran background naturally lends itself to an admiration for the cacao plant; the tree had a presence on my family *finca*, or farm.
>
> —Chef Maribel Leiberman, Marie Belle, New York

late. His journeys throughout the growing regions, along with the reports of scientists and agriculturalists working in these remote areas for many years, cast a hopeful light on the future of chocolate including more education on sustainable farming methods, more stability in crop prices, and even ecotourism to help support the wild forests of these poverty-stricken lands.

Ray Major, head scientist of Artisan Confections (the Hershey's division that runs Scharffen Berger and Dagoba brands, among others), agrees that cacao flourishes with biodiversity, the term scientists use to describe ecosystems like chocolate's natural growing conditions. He told me the story of a farm in Brazil that is a model for the future. It uses rain forest crops to balance the needs of farmers and the needs of the environment. He says, "The true fertility of the rain forest is in the trees and not the soil. To have sustainable and productive farms, farmers need to plant tree crops and, if they are not to be dependent upon the caprices of world commodity prices, the crops need to be diverse and saleable in local markets."

Cacao thrives with bananas, cinnamon, coconut, açaí, passion fruit, pepper, and vanilla, which can be harvested in cacao's off seasons. Together, they create farming opportunities that encourage people of the region to keep old groves intact while planting new trees within them—supporting farmers as well as the rain forest. Perhaps this is chocolate's most unexpected gift to an overpopulated world. But the rigors of cacao farming make this gift a mixed blessing.

the people

Harvesting cacao is no picnic. You trudge through thick bug-infested groves, dodge vines and snakes, and reach for large ripe pods with metal clippers on a stick. You pluck the pods carefully, so as not to damage the trees' ability to generate new ones. You try to avoid getting hit in the head by falling football-sized fruits. Then you lug heavy sacks of pods through the jungle to a spot where you can load them up in a truck. You do all this with a machete strapped to your skin or lodged between your teeth. You drive over bumpy roads with washed-out bridges. When you get back to what amounts to a base

fair trade and organic chocolate companies

In this growing sector of the chocolate business, flavor profiles vary wildly between brands. But all of these companies are committed to a high set of standards for sourcing their beans in an ethical fashion. They also want to educate and engage customers about their processes. Buying their products supports positive ethics.

Alter Eco, www.altereco.com.

Dagoba Organic Chocolate, www.dagobachocolate.com.

Divine Chocolate, www.divinechocolate.com.

Endangered Species Chocolate Company, www.chocolatebar.com.

Equal Exchange, www.equalexchange.com.

Green and Black's Organic, www.greenandblacks.com.

Kallari, www.kallari.com.

Lake Champlain Chocolates, www.lakechamplainchocolates.com.

Newman's Own Organics, www.newmansownorganics.com.

Omanhene Cocoa Bean Company, www.omanhene.com.

Taza Chocolate, www.tazachocolate.com.

Terra Nostra Organic Chocolate, www.terranostrachocolate.com.

Theo Chocolate, www.theochocolate.com.

camp, you open the pods with your machete and scoop out the seeds, hoping monkeys or squirrels or fungus didn't get there first. You have to be quick about opening these pods because if you leave them or their seeds alone for too long, they will rot. Then you have to haul them to their fermenting bins and dump them in. All of this effort is in relentlessly humid, equatorial heat. Slaves and indentured servants assumed the bulk of cacao labor as the colonizing forces of Spain, the Netherlands, England, France, and Belgium took control of the growing regions in the 1700s and 1800s. As with sugar, coffee, and cotton, chocolate's history includes the ugly reality of slavery and its implicit horrors. With the help of slave labor, cocoa beans were shipped, as they are now, to picturesque European countries to be processed under the much more humane conditions of factories, then distributed to the wealthy consuming countries around the world.

In her book *Bitter Chocolate*, journalist Carol Off chronicles the history of slavery in the cacao trade. The practice was eliminated from the cacao-producing system in the early 1900s, yet shocking reports of child labor and slavery from the remote groves of Ivory Coast exploded in 2000. In response to the acute poverty of nearby Mali, rings of child traffickers emerged to send child laborers to the cacao fields of Ivory Coast. A humanitarian and media intervention began, embarrassing and threatening the chocolate industry. Even the biggest, most profit-motivated global food companies shuddered at the possibility that child slaves or indentured servants harvested their crops. The corporations blamed the governments and the governments blamed the corporations; nobody solved the problem. But all agreed the practice needed to stop. The United Nations formed a coalition, the Harkin-Engel Protocol (named after the United States senator and congressman who got involved), to eliminate these conditions. Today the circumstances are better, but not solved. We are a long way from social justice in Africa, and by extension, the growing regions in the world.

The only good news is that chocolate lovers can help.

giving back to chocolate

The best way to help the fragile balance of chocolate's growing conditions and the needs of its people is to educate yourself about labels, environmental initiatives, and humanitarian efforts in the growing regions. Here is a to-do list that can guide you to a mindful approach toward your chocolate.

buy from companies practicing sustainable farming

One of the biggest agricultural challenges in chocolate's future is to reverse farming systems that don't protect the long-term needs of the farmers, the cacao trees, or the rain forest. Some, but not all, chocolate companies invest in sustainable farming methods that help both farmers and crops. Could they, should they, do more to help? Yes, by all accounts, and their track records are checkered at best. You want to support companies with a framework for prosocial and proenvironmental efforts. The following are the most visible companies responding to the humanitarian and conservation issues that face their industry.

Barry Callebaut. By offering the widest range of organic brands of all the big chocolate corporations, Barry Callebaut's support of sustainable farming practices is clear and growing in the right direction.

Cadbury. A recent announcement that England's best-selling candy bar, Cadbury Dairy Milk, will be made exclusively with Fair Trade cocoa beans (see page 82) made Cadbury's prosustainability position very clear.

Hershey's. A prosocial company on many fronts, and "big chocolate" on others, Hershey's initiatives include active environmental stewardship and committed resources toward sustainable farming in conjunction with the World Cocoa Foundation. Hershey's now includes organic and ethically responsible brands Dagoba and Scharffen Berger under the name "Artisan Confections."

Mars, Inc. Philippe Metzger, vice president of sustainability for Mars Western Europe, says: "We invest significant resources to help support the sustainability of the cocoa supply chain—partly because it is linked to our own business success, but also because it is critical to protecting this unique and fragile crop for future generations." Like all corporate chocolate companies, Mars is "big chocolate," very profit

organizations helping chocolate and the growing regions

Equator Initiative, www.EquatorInitiative.org. A United Nations group seeking to reduce poverty and increase sustainable use of biodiversity around the equator, including chocolate's growing regions.

International Red Cross, www.icrc.org/eng. They are in the field working to provide aid to the neediest victims of war and famine, which affect many cacao growers. Descriptions of the relief efforts in specific regions are reported, and online donations are easy to make.

Rainforest Alliance, www.rainforestalliance.com. This organization features an "Adopt-a-Rainforest" program, where donors can contribute to efforts to protect specific people and regions. The cacao farmers of Ecuador are one such group you can support.

Save Africa's Children, www.saveafricaschildren.com. A small group committed to supporting some of the neediest children in the world, the orphans of AIDS in sub-Saharan Africa. Orphanages in Ghana and Ivory Coast, the countries which produce 70 percent of the world's chocolate, are supported by their work.

World Cocoa Foundation, www.worldcocoafoundation.org. This is an active organization devoted to the betterment of the lives of cocoa farmers and sustainable growing practices. Their homepage includes a tab where you can easily contribute online.

driven and controversial on social issues. But their investments, especially in flavanol research, sustainable farming, and bioengineering, are impressive.

buy fair trade

Fair Trade is a humanitarian effort designed to lift farmers out of poverty by investing in the communities, tools, and trees of their trade. Fair Trade (a network of nongovernment organizations, or NGOs) has been successful in helping to regulate the coffee trade, whose farmers, like cacao growers, are vulnerable to the ravages of supply, demand, plant disease, drought, and poverty. Fair Trade guarantees farmers a set price for their crops, even if the commodities market rises higher or lower than that price. In exchange, farmers must join a local cooperative that initiates social improvements, like systems to ensure clean drinking water or organic pest management or education for children. Fair Trade has grown quickly, especially as corporate coffee companies—Starbucks, Peets, and the Coffee Bean & Tea Leaf to name a few—began springing up in every city in the developed world and sought to avoid the public relations trap of exploiting or appearing to exploit farmers. TransFair (the international body that started Fair Trade Certification) cites that bringing awareness to the conditions of farmers in developing countries is one of their main and successfully achieved goals.

Critics contend that Fair Trade is too bureaucratic to help the neediest of the poor. One of Fair Trade's tenets is that agricultural products (in this case, cacao) must be grown organically with no pesticides. Yet many of the impoverished farmers are much too poor to afford pesticides, let alone the fees for joining a co-op or getting certification. Thus, Fair Trade is a certificate process and a community system rather than a direct charity. But it has done more than any other organization to bring to light issues of ethical farming in developing countries. Even with its limitations, Fair Trade is a good beginning in bringing some of the wellness chocolate generates in the developed world back to its roots. Consumer spending on brands with Fair Trade and/or organic labels has established a strong market, and the big companies are convinced of the importance of ethical values, or at least the business they bring.

buy organic

Organic certification is a tricky label for small farmers and consumers alike. The organic produce market is the fastest growing segment of the food service business. For many, the label "organic" connotes quality ingredients, responsible growing conditions, freedom from pesticides, and high-quality food worth a premium price. Yet, as mentioned above, for many small farmers in developing countries, to acquire an organic certification (run by the USDA in the United States) is a prohibitively costly, bureaucratic hurdle. Critics charge that those in the business of marketing the organic label fare much better than those who grow the food.

Strange how benevolent organizations become entangled in aggravating or neglecting the people they hope to empower. No easy solutions exist for the disparities that plague our supplying nations or the problems encountered by those who try to help. Imperfect though it may be, organic certification is a solid stepping stone for the next wave of programs to address the need for pesticide-free, environmentally friendly, socially conscious farming.

make direct donations

You can make a direct contribution to a farm in the country of origin of your favorite chocolate or to the poorest growing region (Madagascar) or to the ones with the most urgent need for rain forest protection (Brazil and Indonesia). How much should you give? How about making a list of the joyful times you indulged your own love of chocolate by ordering a great dessert or impulsively grabbing a candy bar that made your day a little brighter? Assign a donation value for each memory. If you donate a dollar per moment, you will make a contribution that will really, really matter. (See page 81 for specific organizations to support.) Or toss a certificate of donation into a gift basket for a friend, along with a baked goodie and jar of homemade chocolate lotion.

earthy recipes: from chili to cheesecake

These recipes pay homage to the diverse cuisines of chocolate's growing regions. You'll find ingredients native to Mexico, Thailand, Ghana, and Madagascar. As we become aware of the geographic sources of our food, we can celebrate the humble hands that offer chocolate to the world.

chicken with mole negro sauce

Authentic, fiery mole sauces from the southern region of Mexico take days to prepare. This is a relatively quick version of the chunky, spicy, and chocolatey, *mole negro* or "black sauce." To experience the full flavors of peppers, native spices, and fresh chocolate, book a culinary vacation to Oaxaca, Mexico, the Land of Seven Moles, where you can explore a district known as the Trail of Chocolate. In the meantime, get fresh ingredients from your local farmers' market. You can substitute jalepeños for the poblano chiles, but the dark dried ancho and mulato chiles are important to bring the sauce to its characteristic deep chocolate brown. This will make a large batch of sauce designed to thin and use for a meal, then freeze and thaw as needed. **Makes 1 chicken plus 2 cups extra sauce**

Preheat the oven to 350°F. Place the ancho and mulato chiles in a small bowl. Pour boiling water over them and allow them to soften for 15 minutes. Meanwhile, prepare the poblano chile by heating each side under the broiler until the skin turns black. Place the blackened chile on a cutting board, cut off the stem, remove and discard the seeds, and chop coarsely. You'll feel some heat on your hands so be careful not to rub your eyes. Remove the anchos and mulatos from the water, and stem, seed, and chop them as you did the other chiles. Place all the chopped chiles in the bowl of a food processor.

Rinse the chicken in warm water. Remove its giblets and neck, puncture the skin with a fork all around the top, dust it with salt and pepper, then place it on a rack in a baking dish. Place the chicken in the oven for about 1 1/2 hours or until an instant-read thermometer inserted into the thickest part of the thigh reads 165°F.

Meanwhile, scatter the peanuts, almonds, walnuts, pumpkin seeds, sesame seeds, peppercorns, and cloves on

continued

4 dried ancho chiles

1 dried mulato chile

1 poblano chile

1 medium (4- to 5-pound) whole organic chicken

Pinch of kosher salt

Pinch of ground black pepper

1/4 cup roasted, salted peanuts

1/4 cup blanched almonds

1/4 cup walnuts

1/4 cup pumpkin seeds

2 tablespoons sesame seeds

3 whole peppercorns

3 whole cloves

1 pound tomatoes, or 1 (14.5-ounce) can

1 teaspoon ground cinnamon

3 ounces dark chocolate, melted

2 tablespoons dutch-processed, unsweetened cocoa powder

2 corn tortillas

1/4 cup raisins

1/4 cup prunes

3 tablespoons lime juice (approximately 2 limes)

11/2 cups chicken broth

2 tablespoons corn oil

2 cloves garlic, chopped

1 onion, chopped

2 shallots, chopped

1 cup water

2 bunches cilantro sprigs

a baking sheet. Roast them next to the chicken for about 20 minutes, or until they turn dark. Transfer them to the bowl of the food processor with the chiles. Add the tomatoes, cinnamon, chocolate, cocoa powder, tortillas, raisins, prunes, lime juice, and chicken broth. Blend until smooth with a slightly chunky texture from the nuts. Depending on the size of your food processor, you may need to process in two batches. Pour the sauce into a large pot.

Heat the corn oil in a skillet over medium-high heat. Add the garlic and sauté for about 2 minutes, or until it starts to turn light brown. Add the onion and shallots and sauté for about 5 minutes, or until soft. Then add the vegetables to the large pot of sauce. Add the water slowly, stir occasionally, and cook over low heat for about 30 minutes. At any point as the sauce cooks, you can insert an immersion blender to create a smoother texture. Once the sauce simmers, remove the chicken from the oven, cover the top and the inside of the neck cavity with sauce, then return it to the oven to finish cooking. Reserve the remaining sauce for serving, keeping it on very low heat as the chicken finishes cooking.

When the chicken reaches 165°F (about 11/2 hours), the sauce will be dried and blackened. Remove the chicken from the oven, scrape the blackened sauce off, then slice the breast with a sharp knife. Remove the drumsticks and wings if desired. Adjust the thickness of your sauce to taste, thinning it with water as needed. Arrange the slices, wings, and drumsticks on a platter and cover with a stripe of sauce over the center. Garnish with cilantro sprigs.

cocoa chili

Like chocolate, the chile peppers that give chili its name and flavor come from Mexico. By assembling the many ingredients below and allowing them to cook together over low heat, you can easily imagine earlier versions of this Mexican stew (despite a few modern concessions). The cocoa powder adds depth and earthiness to the spicy indigenous flavors. This is a big batch and serves 15 people. You can also freeze it. **Makes 15 cups chili**

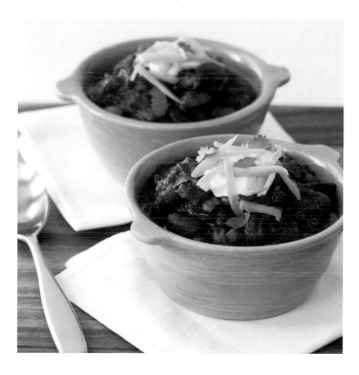

1 tablespoon olive oil

2 cloves garlic, chopped

1 onion, chopped

1 jalapeño or serrano pepper, seeded and chopped

1 bunch scallions, both white and tender green parts, trimmed and chopped

1 pound ground beef (about 80 percent lean)

1 pound ground turkey

2 (28-ounce) cans crushed tomatoes, or 20 fresh tomatoes, peeled, seeded, and chopped

1 (15-ounce or smaller) can kidney beans with liquid

1 (15-ounce or smaller) can pinto beans with liquid

1¹/2 cups spicy salsa

2 tablespoons chili powder

continued

2 tablespoons alkalized or dutched cocoa powder

1 tablespoon ground cumin

1 tablespoon kosher salt

1 tablespoon ground black pepper

1 teaspoon hot sauce, or more, such as Tabasco or Tapatió

1 large bunch fresh cilantro, chopped

1/2 cup grated Cheddar cheese

1/2 cup sour cream

Heat the olive oil in a large skillet over medium heat. Add the garlic and sauté for a minute or two until the edges start to brown. Add the onion, chile, and scallions and sauté for about 2 minutes, or until they soften. Add the ground beef and turkey and cook for about 8 minutes, or until brown. Drain off the excess fat and transfer the mixture to a big pot. Add the tomatoes, kidney and pinto beans, salsa, chili powder, cocoa powder, cumin, salt, pepper, and hot sauce. Allow the mixture to simmer over low heat for about 20 minutes. Taste and adjust the seasonings. If you have an immersion blender, you can use it here to create a smoother chili. Either way, allow the chili to simmer over low heat for another 30 minutes. Add half of the cilantro and reserve the rest to use as garnish for individual servings.

Serve hot with the cheese, sour cream, and the remaining cilantro on top.

milk chocolate dulce de leche

Many recipes for this Latin American caramel sauce suggest using a can of sweetened condensed milk. But if you make *dulce de leche* from scratch, as this recipe specifies, you'll get a delicate sweetness from cooked sugar and fresh milk no canned product can ever match. It is very easy but takes a long time—about 1 1/2 hours, even though all you have to do is give it an occasional stir. Here's the trick: choose a time when you'll be in the kitchen awhile—maybe a weekend afternoon or a night you are making another slow-cooked sauce. This version, untraditionally, is flavored with milk chocolate. Serve over ice cream or pound cake. Makes 3 cups sauce

Stir together the milk, sugar, baking soda, vanilla bean pod and seeds, and salt in a large saucepan. Bring to a boil over medium heat; the mixture will bubble up high. Stir and turn the heat to low. Then let the sauce simmer. Skim it occasionally with a strainer to remove the milk scum, and stir the bottom of the pan with a wooden spoon or heatproof spatula to make sure the milk solids don't scorch. After about an hour, remove the vanilla bean pod. The sauce will slowly turn light brown, reduce, and turn honey-colored. You want it to reach a dark amber color but still be pourable. The total cooking time is about 1 1/2 to 2 hours. For a thin, sweet sauce, 1 1/2 hours will do it. If you like a thicker texture, keep cooking all the way to 2 hours. Once you're reached an amber color and a suitably thick texture, take the sauce off the heat and allow it to cool for 5 minutes.

Put the milk chocolate in a small bowl. Pour the *dulce de leche* mixture over it and stir until the sauce is smooth. Serve immediately or store in the refrigerator for later use (such as making Fudgey Hearts of Darkness, page 36).

Chocolate Choices
Endangered Species milk chocolate, Scharffen Berger Milk Chocolate, or Valrhona Jivara Lactée

4 cups whole milk

1 1/2 cups sugar

1/2 teaspoon baking soda

1 vanilla bean, scraped and seeded

1/2 teaspoon kosher salt

3 ounces milk chocolate, finely chopped

fair trade mocha lemon cheesecake

Blending Fair Trade coffee with Fair Trade cocoa allows us to support those who serve the world coffee and chocolate. It also helps us celebrate the classic European flavor combination of coffee and chocolate, mixed here as you might find them in an Italian café, with tangy mascarpone cheese and lemon. To make the cookie crumbs for the crust, see the recipe for Chocolate Sugar Dough (page 132) or buy plain cookies (like Pepperidge Farm Chocolate Chessman). Toss about twenty cookies of either type in the blender, pulse two or three times, and you will have dark chocolate cookie crumbs. You'll need a cheesecake or springform pan, and most grocery store versions of this work fine. When the cake is baked and chilled, release the latch, slice, and serve. Be sure to clean your knife with a warm wet towel for each slice. **Makes 1 (9-inch) cheesecake**

Chocolate Choices

Fair Trade cocoa powder, such as Equal Exchange or Green & Black's

Crust

1/2 cup chocolate cookie crumbs, plus 1 cup for garnish (optional)

1/4 cup unsweetened cocoa powder

1/2 cup crushed pecans

2 tablespoons Fair Trade espresso or coffee beans, such as Green Mountain Coffee or Grounds for Change, coarsely chopped

3 tablespoons unsalted butter, melted

Preheat the oven to 350°F.

To make the crust, combine the cookie crumbs, cocoa powder, pecans, espresso beans, and butter in a small bowl and mix to form a paste. Be sure to save 1 cup of cookie crumbs to use as garnish if you'd like chocolate crumbs on the sides of the cake. Scoop the mixture into a standard 9-inch wide and 3-inch deep cheesecake pan (if using a one-piece pan, place a circle of parchment paper in the bottom first; a springform pan doesn't require it) and pat in firmly to form an even crust just on the bottom, not up the sides. Cover with plastic wrap and set in the refrigerator.

To make the batter, in the bowl of an electric mixer fitted with the paddle attachment, blend the cream cheese on medium speed until it is completely smooth. Stop the mixer, add the mascarpone cheese, sour cream, and sugar and continue to mix on low speed until smooth. Add the eggs one at a time and beat until incorporated. Next, add the lemon juice, lemon oil, espresso, vanilla, and salt and beat until smooth.

Remove the crust from the refrigerator and remove the plastic wrap. Pour the batter into the pan. Create a water bath by placing the cheesecake pan in a bigger baking pan and gently pouring room temperature water into the bigger pan until it reaches about 1 inch up the side of the cheesecake pan.

Bake for 1 hour and 15 minutes, or until it is lightly browned on top. You'll need two good pot holders to get the cake out. Carefully pull it up and out of the water bath, then to a safe spot to cool. Carefully remove the pan of hot water and dump it out in the sink. Allow the cheesecake to cool for about 1 hour, then place it in the refrigerator. It needs about 4 hours in the refrigerator to fully set up.

Before serving, release the cake from its pan. For a springform pan, run a paring knife along the inside of the pan, then slowly release the hinge on the outside of the pan. For a one-piece pan, run a paring knife along the inside of the pan, then cover the pan with a piece of parchment paper and then a sheet pan. Flip the pans so the cheesecake releases onto the parchment-covered sheet pan. Remove the parchment paper the cake baked on. The cake will be chocolate side up. Place a serving plate over the chocolate side of the cheesecake, the flip it again so that it is chocolate side down. Smooth any dings on the top with a hot dinner knife. Garnish the cake by pressing chocolate cookie crumbs on the sides with your palms. Add a few espresso beans, candied lemon peels, or a few curls of shaved chocolate on top.

Batter

3 (8-ounce) packages cream cheese, at room temperature

1 (8-ounce) package mascarpone cheese, at room temperature

1/2 cup sour cream, at room temperature

1 cup sugar

3 large eggs

2 tablespoons fresh lemon juice

1 tablespoon lemon oil, or finely grated zest of 1 whole lemon

2 tablespoons strong brewed espresso or coffee

1 tablespoon vanilla extract

1 teaspoon kosher salt

Espresso beans, candied lemon peel, or chocolate curls, for garnish

new world pumpkin spice cake with chocolate glaze

This moist cake combines the fruits, nuts, and spices from the New World that the Spanish conquistadores discovered in 1508. Chocolate was part of this Mesoamerican tableau. Brown sugar and ginger arrived much later, but this cake pays homage to the riches of the original jungles and river valleys.   Makes 1 (9-inch) bundt cake

Chocolate Choices

Nestlé Crunch (which adds puffed rice crunch to the glaze), Cadbury Roast Almond chocolate bar (which adds the crunch of almond pieces), or Endangered Species milk chocolate

Cake

2 cups cake flour

1 tablespoon baking soda

1 teaspoon kosher salt

1 teaspoon ground cinnamon

1/2 teaspoon ground nutmeg

1/2 teaspoon ground cloves

1 scant teaspoon grated fresh ginger

4 large eggs

2 cups firmly packed light brown sugar

Preheat the oven to 350°F. Generously grease a standard Bundt cake pan with oil or butter, then dust flour on the greased inside of the pan. Fluted Bundt pans, especially, need a lot of grease for the cake to release.

To make the cake, sift together the flour, baking soda, salt, cinnamon, nutmeg, cloves, and ginger. Set aside.

In a large bowl, beat together the eggs and brown sugar with a whisk until light and fluffy. Add the vegetable oil and pumpkin puree and stir until smooth. Add half of the flour mixture and mix until it is absorbed. Then add the rest of the flour mixture followed by the vanilla, rum, cocoa nibs, and pecans. Switch to a rubber spatula to stir the mixture until smooth. Use the rubber spatula to scoop the batter into the prepared pan.

Bake for about 45 minutes, or until a toothpick or bamboo skewer inserted into the center of the cake comes out with just a few crumbs, not batter. Allow the cake to cool in the pan to room temperature before inverting in onto a wire rack.

To make the glaze, combine the chocolate, butter, milk, corn syrup, and salt in a stainless steel bowl over a saucepan of simmering water over medium heat and stir as the ingredients melt together. Pour the glaze over the cake after the cake has cooled to room temperature. You'll have extra glaze left over, which you can pour into the center of the cake or save to serve with plated slices.

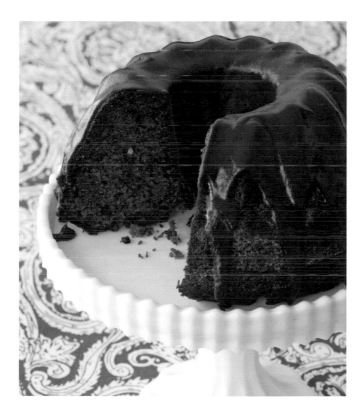

1 cup vegetable oil

1 1/2 cups cooked pumpkin puree or 1 (15-ounce) can

1 tablespoon vanilla extract

1 tablespoon dark rum

1/2 cup cocoa nibs

1 cup pecans, broken into small pieces

Glaze

8 ounces milk chocolate, finely chopped

1/4 cup (1/2 stick) unsalted butter

2 tablespoons milk

1 tablespoon light corn syrup

1 teaspoon kosher salt

tropical tree banana nut muffins

Banana leaves gracefully cover cocoa beans in their fermenting bins where the beans develop their extraordinary flavor. Roadside farm stands in chocolate's growing regions offer a jumble of bananas, cinnamon sticks, plantains, cacao pods, walnuts, vanilla beans, and coconuts, all from trees of the tropics. For that extra earth-friendly touch, use muffin or cupcake liners made with unbleached, eco-friendly paper.

Makes 12 large muffins

1 cup all-purpose flour

1 cup whole-wheat flour

2 teaspoons baking powder

1/2 teaspoon baking soda

1 teaspoon kosher salt

1/2 teaspoon ground cinnamon or grated from a cinnamon stick

1/2 teaspoon ground nutmeg

1/2 teaspoon ground ginger

1 cup (2 sticks) unsalted cold butter

1/2 cup firmly packed dark brown sugar

2 large eggs

3 ripe bananas, sliced

1/2 cup toasted coconut (preferably ribbon or sliced coconut, lightly chopped)

1/4 cup sour cream

1 teaspoon fresh lemon juice

1/2 cup broken walnuts

8 ounces semisweet chocolate chips, or 1 cup dark chocolate pieces

3 ounces milk chocolate, grated with a vegetable peeler

Preheat the oven to 350°F. Lightly grease a 12-cup muffin pan and insert muffin liners in each cavity.

Sift together the all-purpose and whole wheat flours, baking powder, baking soda, salt, cinnamon, nutmeg, and ginger.

In the bowl of an electric mixer fitted with the paddle attachment, cream the butter on low speed until it is soft. Add the brown sugar and beat at medium speed until fluffy. Add the eggs, one at a time, beating well after each addition. Next add the bananas, coconut, sour cream, and lemon juice and mix briefly until they are incorporated. Stop the mixer and slowly add half the flour and spice mixture. Mix a little on slow, then add the rest and mix until incorporated. Take the bowl off the mixer, and fold in the walnuts and chocolate chips. Use a ladle to scoop the batter into the muffin cups.

Bake at 350°F for about 25 minutes. The muffins should rise in a domed shape and are ready when a toothpick inserted into the center of a muffin comes out clean with a few crumbs but no batter. When the muffins are done, take them out of the oven and sprinkle over each one the grated milk chocolate, which will melt as a topping. Remove them from the pan with the wrapper still attached and serve on a platter with fresh fruit.

culinary classes

Want to learn chocolate work from the best? Check out these professional programs.

Burdick's Chocolate Cooking School. Walpole, New Hampshire. www.burdickchocolate.com/chocolate_cooking_school.asp.

Barry Callebaut's Chocolate Academy. Chicago, Illinois, and International. www.barry-callebaut.com.

The Culinary Institute of America. Hyde Park, New York, and St. Helena, California. www.ciachef.edu.

French Culinary Institute at the International Culinary Center. New York, New York. www.frenchculinary.com.

Le Cordon Bleu Schools. North America, www.lecordonbleuschoolsusa.com, and International, www.cordonbleu.edu.

Lenôtre. Paris, France. www.lenotre.fr.

The Notter School of Pastry Arts. Orlando, Florida. www.notterschool.com.

Richardson Researches, Inc. University of California, Davis. www.richres.com.

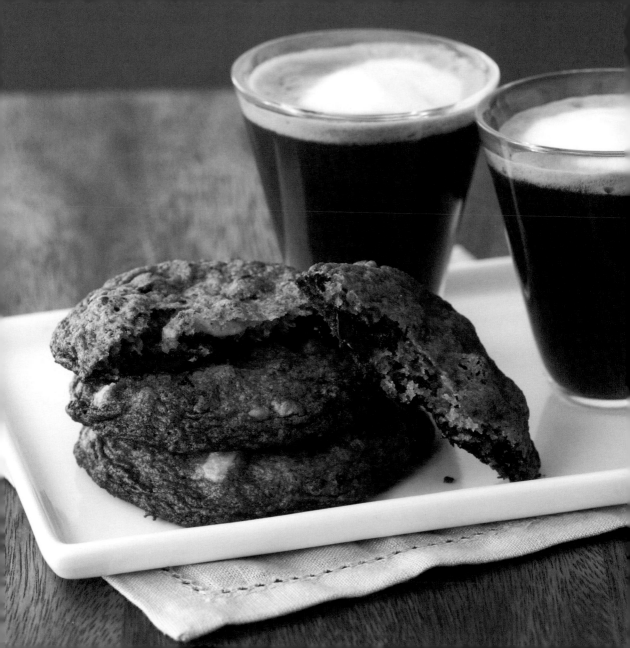

nutty, nibby chocolate chip cookies

These chocolate chip cookies have nuts and cocoa nibs, which give them an earthy crunch. Be sure to chill the dough before you scoop it out so the cookies will keep their shape as they bake. **Makes about 24 medium cookies**

Sift together the flour, baking soda, and salt and set aside. Cream the butter in the bowl of an electric mixer fitted with the paddle attachment at low speed. Add the granulated and brown sugars and mix until the mixture becomes light and fluffy. Slowly add the wheat germ, then the eggs, one at a time. Mix until smooth. Stop the mixer and add the flour mixture slowly, then resume mixing at low speed. Remove the bowl from the mixer and fold in the vanilla, chocolate chips, cocoa nibs, pecans, and Brazil nuts with a large spatula. Mix just until all the ingredients are incorporated. Chill the dough in the bowl covered in plastic wrap in the refrigerator for 30 minutes.

Preheat the oven to 350°F. Line two baking sheets with parchment paper.

Use an ice cream scoop or two large spoons to form the cookie dough into uniform shapes and place on the baking sheet about 1 inch apart. Bake the cookies for 10 to 12 minutes, until light golden brown. When they are done, remove the baking sheet from the oven and allow the cookies to cool for about 5 minutes before moving them to a plate.

2 cups all-purpose flour

1 tablespoon baking soda

1 teaspoon kosher salt

1 cup (2 sticks) unsalted cold butter

1/2 cup granulated sugar

1 cup firmly packed light brown sugar

2 tablespoons toasted wheat germ

2 large eggs

1 tablespoon vanilla extract

12 ounces chocolate chips or semisweet chocolate, finely chopped

1/2 cup chopped cocoa nibs

1/2 cup broken pecans

1/2 cup chopped Brazil nuts or macadamias

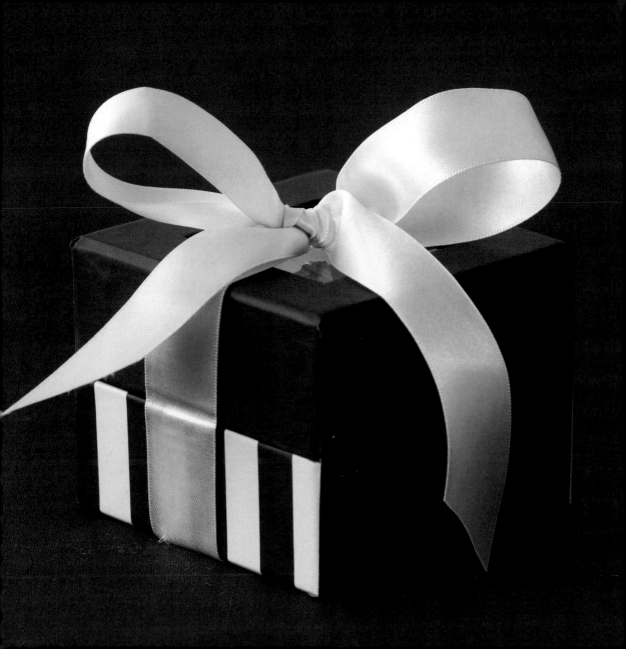

4 share the love

✦

THE GIFT OF CHOCOLATE

You don't get a name like "food of the gods" for nothing. In the dramatic legends of Mesoamerica from about 1000 C.E., a feather-headed serpent god named Quetzalcoatl ruled agriculture and wisdom. He gave the cacao tree as a gift to farmers in the fields to show his respect for them and thus to all mankind. Then the goddess of love, Xochiquetzal, adorned the tree with delicate white flowers. From each white flower grew a pod, and from each pod sprung cacao beans, bringing the fruitful gift of chocolate to people of the world. When you hear the phrase "the food of the gods" (its official name, *Theobroma cacao*, was assigned by Swedish botanist Carl Linnaeus in 1876, noticeably combining Greek and Aztec languages), you'll understand that chocolate has been considered a divine and sacred gift for thousands of years.

Elaine Gonzalez, author and specialist in chocolate and the cultures of Latin American, explained the complexities of the legends of the gods to me. For the ancients, the cacao pod represented the human heart and chocolate represented human blood. Particularly in the Aztec culture, humans were sacrificed to the gods with the heart sliced out of the body, still beating. This was thought to please Huitzilopochtli, a sun god, and generate his good will toward another day. Chocolate was a drink for kings and noblemen—leaders of these religious ceremonies. Further, cocoa beans were a form of currency in the trade of the Maya and the Aztec and probably the Olmec. Cocoa was a valuable part of their religious and commercial cultures. Growers in Mexico today understand this legacy and associate it with chocolate's enduring power to generate love, wealth, and power.

Another historian offers insight into chocolate's spirituality. Sophie Coe, late wife of Michael D. Coe, professor emeritus of anthropology at Yale, was a passionate scholar and food historian, happily at work on her chocolate history book when she died. As a gift to her, Michael completed *The True History of Chocolate*, a comprehensive and authoritative book based on her research. The authors infused their work with a spirit larger than the considerably large history of chocolate. Their book contains the double gifts of chocolate and love and became the most respected book on chocolate history ever produced.

Chocolate has evolved as an important part of our contemporary gift-giving. It embodies romantic love, familial love, the celebration of seasons, and self-indulgence in all the best ways possible.

the chocolate-covered holidays

We connect with others and enrich ourselves through gift-giving. Because of chocolate's unique ability to please adults and children, its status as an affordable luxury, and its capacity to provide simple, sensuous pleasure, chocolate is one of the most popular gifts in the Western world.

Giving thanks to gods and goddesses for food is a common thread in every major religion of the world throughout time, particularly Buddhism, Christianity, Judaism, and the polytheistic religions practiced by Greeks, Romans, and Mesoamericans. Early Christian missionaries developed a pattern of "Christianizing" pagan holidays—keeping the schedule and familiar traditions of the sacrificial pagan festivals, but changing the intentions and iconography to reflect Christian beliefs. Over time, dependably pleasing chocolate became a regular feature in holiday traditions. Gifts, including chocolate, symbolize religious, social, psychological, and romantic wellness. Despite how radically our belief systems have changed since the days of the Aztec gods, chocolate remains a universal gift of love.

chocolate and the arts: literature

Roald Dahl. Perhaps the most famous novel about chocolate is *Charlie and the Chocolate Factory*, in which a young boy longs for access to the mysterious local chocolate factory.*

Charles Dickens. Disdain for the aristocracy bubbles up in *A Tale of Two Cities* when the elaborate chocolate preparation practiced by a holy man becomes a symbol of foolish excess.

Laura Esquivel. *Like Water for Chocolate* explores the spirituality of food and cooking brought to life by a girl's romantic longings and strict sense of family duty.*

Gustave Flaubert. Madame Bovary, the pretentious and beguiling heroine in Flaubert's most renowned novel, is prescribed medicinal chocolate by her doting husband to soothe her luxury-craving soul.

Joanne Harris. *Chocolat* measures the mystical power of chocolate and sensuality against the restrictive rules of the Catholic Church in rural France.*

Ernest Hemingway. In the short story "A Way You'll Never Be," a soldier proves he is American by referring to his stash of chocolate bars, a common wartime ration.

James Joyce. The two Dublin heroes of the 1922 novel *Ulysses* are the old, wary Leopold Bloom and the young, injured Stephen Dedalus. When Leopold makes Stephen a cup of cocoa and Stephen notes his hospitality, the exchange symbolizes a crucial moment of rescue for both characters. Joyce calls this vehicle "the creature cocoa."

Marcel Proust. In *Rememberance of Things Past*, Proust's semiautobiographical narrator delights in hot cocoa, chocolate cream, and gateaux.

Leo Tolstoy. Russian leading lady Anna Karenina is fiendishly bittersweet. Despite her self-ishness, her strongest moments of grace occur when she shows affection toward her son. When she procures European chocolate for him, a status symbol in the Russian aristocracy, we recognize it as a meaningful gift of motherly love.

*Watch the film, too!

halloween

Halloween is the holiday of American mini candy bars—more are sold at this time of year than any other. For those of us who love chocolate—all chocolate—Halloween is a race to swallow up the silly candy of our childhoods while digging up as many new treasures as a jumbo orange jack-o'-lantern bucket will hold.

You know the icons of American Halloween: ghosts, zombies, bats, witches, and vampires. These ghouls date back to autumnal Celtic fire festivals (also known as Samhain) that began around 500 B.C.E. The Celts sought to share the riches of their autumn harvest with their departed ones, in hopes of nourishing journeys through the afterlife. After the Romans took over the Celtic lands of Ireland, England, and parts of Europe, the fire festivals eventually merged with the Roman Catholic All Souls Day, a late October time to honor the souls of the noble departed. Despite generations of changes in religious thinking, the ghostliness of ancient pagan festivals and a Roman celebration of the dead remain remarkably intact and spooky as our very own Halloween. The only thing missing from the ancient rites was chocolate, which hadn't made its way to Europe yet. To add chocolate to this mix of holiday traditions, we needed Mexican influence.

Mexico's El Día de los Muertos (Day of the Dead) is similar to Halloween as a convergence of pagan and Catholic religious traditions. But here, the same symbols of death have a chocolate twist. Smiling skeletons line cake shop windows; bright marigolds and masks are carried through cemeteries in the southwestern United States and Mexico on November 1 to 2, and revelers place cups of hot chocolate, bread, and sugar cakes out to attract and nourish the ghosts of their loved ones. This is a colorful, macabre celebration. The All Soul's Day of the Spanish settlers merged with an ancient Aztec harvest festival similar to that of the Celts. Residue of chocolate has been found on bowls that were buried inside the tombs of Mesoamerican kings and high priests three thousand years ago to nourish them on their journeys to the netherworld. Clearly, Mexico has been serving a Halloween special of death and chocolate for a very long time.

christmas and hanukkah

Today's winter holidays bring an avalanche of chocolate goodies. Advent calendars pop open with chocolate, stockings bulge with chocolate Santas, manufacturers churn out elaborately wrapped gift boxes with ornate bows. The most traditional Christmas cakes, bûche de Nöel in Europe and the yule log in England, are chocolate flavored inside and out. In ancient times, all northern pre-Christian cultures celebrated the winter solstice with light festivals. Fires marked the passing of the long days of winter. That is why Christmas trees, yule logs, tree lights, and candles are so central to our modern celebrations of Christmas. Hanukkah, coincidentally a winter holiday with triumph over pagan theology at its core, has also evolved as a chocolate-touched holiday.

Today, giving chocolate gelt, or money, on Hanukkah is a blessing to children for success. This gelt takes the form of gold- and silver-wrapped chocolate coins. Dreidel games and parties often end with a prize—a bag of chocolate coins. Try being a grown-up at a Hanukkah party and not pocketing a few of those coins! Sometimes, both Hanukkah and Christmas seem like Festivals of Chocolate.

valentine's day

In his *New York Times Magazine* article tracing the history of St. Valentine's Day back to fertility rituals of Eros in ancient Greece and Luperces in ancient Rome, my father-in-law, Jason Epstein, explained how Valentine's Day "conveys a giggling air of carnality and the uncertain promise of raffish coupling." Valentine's Day celebrations stubbornly include fertility symbols: "today's chocolate boxes in the shape of inverted bottoms." You'll never look at a heart-shaped box the same way! Every year, as the days lengthen and animals begin their mating, so we celebrate Valentine's Day with flowers, cards, and chocolate booty boxes. The Greeting Card Association estimates that approximately one billion valentines are sent each year worldwide, making the day the second largest card-sending holiday of the year, behind Christmas. Children participate by sending cards or candies to schoolmates they appreciate, and adults participate by having romantic dinners with rich desserts, giving romantic gifts, sending cards, buying flowers, and, of course, splurging on chocolates in extravagant heart-shaped boxes. Chocolate is associated with this holiday beginning in childhood, and as a child grows into an adult, the subtext may change but the happiness chocolate evokes on Valentine's Day remains the same.

a chocolate wedding

White weddings have held court long enough. Consider making room for your real true love at your wedding: CHOCOLATE.

Cake. Make a Gift of the Gods Chocolate Cake with Sugar Islands Chocolate Buttercream. Use Dark Chocolate Plastique for decorations.

Cocktails. Crème de cacao martinis or Champagne, served with green grapes and white chocolate truffles.

The Menu. Not every dish needs to be drenched in chocolate. Instead, every course should offer a new variation on the chocolate theme. The salad course can include a splash of chocolate vinaigrette, the meat course can be drizzled with a chocolate mole sauce, and chocolate mousse can be served with the coffee or tea (or mochas).

The Favors. Go for small favor boxes with a lot of flare from wedding supply vendors. Then choose top quality chocolates to put inside. Your local artisan chocolatier can also design chocolates and packaging to match your color scheme.

Easter is one of the busiest seasons for chocolatiers. Chocolate Easter bunnies and baskets filled with candy eggs fill the shops. But why don't we celebrate with chocolate palm leaves or crosses? Easter, too, is a combination of ancient fertility rites and Christian religion. In the agricultural societies of pre-Christian Europe, if the days didn't shorten and the sun didn't warm the fields enough for plants to grow and yield, you would be hungry. If your animals did not mate and thrive, you would be even hungrier. Once the calendar moved past the fertility rites of February, wonderful things happened. Baby chicks and baby bunnies! So at Easter, we celebrate not just the Resurrection of Christ but also the arrival of spring, chickens, rabbits, chocolate Easter eggs, and chocolate Easter bunnies. To give Easter chocolate to children is to celebrate all the forces of life that created them.

birthdays: how to make a great birthday cake

We don't know who baked the very first birthday cake, but we know the tradition evolved in Western Europe and the United States in the 1800s. What makes a great birthday cake? Many home bakers buy cake mixes at the supermarket hoping to save time and guarantee good results. But the most you can ever hope for from a boxed cake is mediocrity. Instead, take the plunge and bake a cake from scratch. If you can use a cake mix, you can bake a cake from scratch. What's more, you'll be able to create a cake with personality—a cake with fresh ingredients and deep flavors.

This book offers simple flavor choices for cakes: deep, dark chocolate or velvety vanilla. You can load plenty of different chocolate icings on top of either one— here you'll find four great choices. After you decide on your cake and icing, take a moment to think through the design and all the things you'll need. If you want to decorate your cake with flowers, such as those made from marzipan (available in supermarket or gourmet food stores' baking sections) or white chocolate roses (see page 130), you'll need to pull those ingredients together first so you can work on them while the cake is baking. If you want toasted nuts on the side of your cake, toast them in advance so they'll have time to cool. If you want chocolate icing rosettes on top (and who wouldn't?), plan to make a double batch of icing. These kinds of decisions are part of a pastry chef's and/or birthday cake baker's *mise en place*.

Most pastry chefs prefer to bake the cake one day and make the icing and assemble it all the next day. I resisted this approach at first. Two days to make a cake? But, in fact, the two-day plan eliminates stress. If I need a cake for a Saturday night party, I'll make the cake Friday night. If I'm having a good time, I'll go ahead and make the icing and decorations, too. On Saturday morning, I'll focus on getting the icing to its correct temperature, assembling the cake, and decorating it. Since I usually work with buttercream, I'll need to chill the icing so that it holds its texture or heat it up a little if it is too stiff to spread. These unpredictable variations (often related to room temperature, humidity, or interruptions) are the things that stress you out if you rush and try and do the whole job the day the birthday cake is to be presented.

Once you've baked your cake, made the icing, and perfected the decorations, the steps are: (1) assemble and ice it, and (2) decorate it. To ice a two-layer cake, use an offset spatula. You'll want to spread a generous layer of icing on the first layer of cake. Then put the second layer on top, with the bottom side up since it is usually flatter. Apply a "crumb coat," a thin layer of icing over this assembly of the two layers. (It's called a crumb coat because the inevitable cake crumbs that fall from the cake will stick to it and not mess up your final icing coat. It also provides stability by holding the two layers together.) Then chill it for a half hour. Next, ice the cake with a top coat. Now you are ready to decorate.

No matter how shaky your pastry bag skills are, they will improve with practice. Pastry bags and tips are available at most kitchen stores and crafts stores, plus you can use a sealable plastic storage bag in a pinch. Use your extra icing to create a border of rosettes, or keep it simple and do several icing rosettes on top of the cake. You can also use nuts, cookie crumbs, or candy. When in doubt, keep it simple. Add just a few touches.

Inevitably, you will face the Happy Birthday Challenge. You've got to be able to write "Happy Birthday" in cursive, using melted chocolate in a pastry bag or plastic storage bag with a tiny hole in the corner. This, my friends, takes practice. So practice

nix on the cake mix

Tempting, isn't it, that box of cake mix with the voluptuous slice seducing you from the grocery store shelf? Will your cake look like that? Perfect, shiny, chiseled? Don't be fooled! That cake is on steroids! Cake mix packaging photos are retouched and retooled by a team of marketing people, sometimes even produced with wax and shaving cream to hold up better under studio lights. The mix itself is sullied with preservatives and additives. Nobody wants to eat those things. Cake mix does not really save you any time because there are only two time-consuming tasks involved in making a cake: shopping for the ingredients and searching for the pans. If you are considering buying a box of cake mix, you are already in the grocery store. All you need to do is move down the aisle for a bag of unbleached flour, some sugar, cocoa, and baking powder. Make a quick stop for eggs, milk, butter, and cream and you are on your way to a far superior cake.

Searching for your pans, measuring cups, and measuring spoons in the back of your cabinets is a task you have to do anyway if you work with a mix. If you don't have a mixer at home, buy a big bowl, a big whisk, and some cake pans, and you will make your cake by hand, just as the famous pastry chefs of royal courts did in the Age of Enlightenment.

on a sheet of aluminum foil or parchment paper. If you are a first timer, practice five times, and you'll be ready to approach your cake. Center the word "Happy" on the upper third of the cake top, put "Birthday" right below it, right in the center, then have a little fun with your loved one's name.

cakes for kids

Try Very Vanilla Cake for Chocolate Lovers (page 112) and Cocoa Chantilly Cream (page 117). You won't overwhelm little kids with too much chocolate richness, but you will offer them chocolate flavor in a sweet icing. Use Dark Chocolate Plastique (page 134) like Play-Doh and let them help you make decorations the day before. For older kids and teens, ask them what they want their cake to look like. You are bound to get a strong opinion.

cakes for the 20s

Chocolate lovers in their 20s can handle the good stuff. Try Gift of the Gods Chocolate Cake (page 115) with Sugar Islands Chocolate Buttercream (page 119). Use dark, bold chocolate in both recipes.

cakes for the 30s

I like a cake layer for each decade for people in their 30s. Use one layer of chocolate cake, one layer of vanilla, one layer of chocolate—a triple decade layer cake. Make a Gift of the Gods Chocolate Cake (page 115), then a Very Vanilla Cake for Chocolate Lovers (page 112). Layer them with Cocoa Chantilly Cream (page 117), an easy icing to make (which makes up for the fact that you've just made two cakes). That will leave you one spare layer of vanilla cake you can freeze and serve with fruit and a sauce (such as Sugarplum Sauce, page 64) for an impromptu dessert down the road.

cakes for the 40s

Time for a simple, elegant European-style cake to celebrate the accomplished person turning 40 or beyond. Try the Gift of the Gods Chocolate Cake (page 115), which gives you a sturdy, two-layer cake. Put the first layer on a cake plate or sturdy paper plate. Use Cocoa Chantilly Cream (page 117) in the center with chopped seasonal fruit like peaches or strawberries. Put on the next layer of chocolate cake, then glaze the whole cake with the shine of Glaze of the Gods (page 118).

cakes for the 50s

Make a Very Vanilla Cake for Chocolate Lovers (page 112) and ice with a Sweet Bittersweet Ganache (page 120). Then focus on decorations that celebrate who they are and what they love. If they love purple, load the cake with purple flowers made from White Chocolate Plastique (page 135). If they love movies, make cinema reels and a box of popcorn out of marzipan, White Chocolate Plastique (page 135), or Dark Chocolate Plastique (page 134).

cakes for the 60s

Make cupcakes, because sixty-year-olds appreciate the reminder that you're never too old, using either Very Vanilla Cake for Chocolate Lovers (page 118) or Gift of the Gods Chocolate Cake (page 115). Make the batter as the recipes instruct, then pour it into muffin tins lined with cupcake liners. Bake them for about 25 minutes instead of the 40 minutes or so most cakes require. Ice the cupcakes with Cocoa Chantilly Cream on page 117 (you can include $1/2$ teaspoon of peppermint extract), dust them with cocoa powder, then add fresh mint leaves and candles on each one.

cakes for the specials

Anybody 70 or older is special. Try a childlike cake that brings them sweet memories of their early days. Make Very Vanilla Cake for Chocolate Lovers (page 118) topped by Sugar

don't forget *your* birthday

You can spend the week before your birthday wondering whether someone is planning a party for you, or you can literally take matters into your own hands. Make yourself a birthday cake. It doesn't have to be a big one. But it has to be one of your favorites. If you are alone on your birthday, you've got something to share with a friend of your choosing. If your friends come through and pull a party together, you have a cake to take along or bring home when it's all done.

Islands Chocolate Buttercream (page 119). Decorate it with the prettiest, most birthday cake-ish roses you can make (White Chocolate Plastique, page 135).

gifting recipes: from cupcakes to white chocolate roses

These recipes are all designed to make and give as gifts. Carefully crafted chocolate brings heartwarming accompaniments: an aura of mystery, sensuous power, memories of childhood, fun, and flavor. In this section, you'll find two cakes and four icings, and they can be mixed and matched as you like. You'll also find cookies, cakes, and candies that travel well and will delight the gift recipient with the power of chocolate.

very vanilla cake for chocolate lovers

This is a moist, fragrant cake with a soft, strong crumb. Its flavors hold up well with chocolate. Use it with Cocoa Chantilly Cream (page 117) for subtle chocolate flavor, or use Sugar Islands Chocolate Buttercream (page 119) for the big bang of chocolate and vanilla together. **Makes 2 (8-inch) cake layers**

3 1/2 cups cake flour

2 tablespoons baking powder

1 teaspoon kosher salt

1 cup (2 sticks) cold unsalted butter

2 cups sugar

1 tablespoon vanilla extract

1 cup whole or 2% milk

8 large egg whites, at room temperature

Preheat the oven to 350°F. Prepare two cake pans (8 inches in diameter, 2 inches deep) by lightly spraying the bottoms and sides with cooking spray. Cut out circles of parchment paper to fit on the bottom of each pan. The paper should be flat, not inching up the sides of the pan. Set the pans aside.

Sift together the cake flour, baking powder, and salt in a bowl and stir with a whisk, then set aside.

In the bowl of an electric mixer fitted with the paddle attachment, cream the butter at low speed until it is soft and fluffy. Switch to the whisk attachment, increase the speed to medium, and slowly add the sugar. Meanwhile, add the vanilla to the milk. Stop the mixer and add half of the milk mixture (it's worth stirring it a little by hand here so that it doesn't splash all over your kitchen), then mix on low until it is incorporated. Next, add half of the flour mixture and mix slowly. Repeat the process by adding the rest of the milk mixture, stirring slowly, then adding the rest of the flour. Remove from the mixer and use a large rubber spatula to stir until smooth. Transfer this batter to a large bowl and set aside. This is your vanilla batter.

Thoroughly rinse and dry your mixer bowl and whisk attachment. Then put the egg whites in the bowl and mix on low at first, then increase speed to medium. After a few minutes, the egg whites will hold a medium peak. Fold the whipped egg whites into the batter in thirds with a large rubber spatula, gently folding the batter after each addition. Pour the completed cake batter evenly into the prepared cake pans.

Bake for 35 to 40 minutes. The top of the cake will bubble then rise up and turn golden brown. When a toothpick inserted in the center comes out clean, with no batter, remove from the oven and allow the cakes to cool on a rack to room temperature. You'll notice that the tops deflate a little, but that won't matter in the finished product since those tops will become the bottoms. Allow the cakes to cool to room temperature. Remove the cake layers by using a paring knife to gently cut the cake from the sides of the pan. Take a cake circle or sturdy paper plate, and place it over the pan. Invert the cake onto the plate and remove the parchment circle the cake baked on. Repeat this process for the other cake layer. Ice the first layer with the icing of your choice, with about 1/2 inch of icing on top. Place the second layer onto the cake with the bottom side up, which will give you a flat, undomed top. Ice the whole cake thinly (this is a crumb coat to stabilize the cake and hold the crumbs in place), chill it for at least 20 minutes, then apply a final coat of icing.

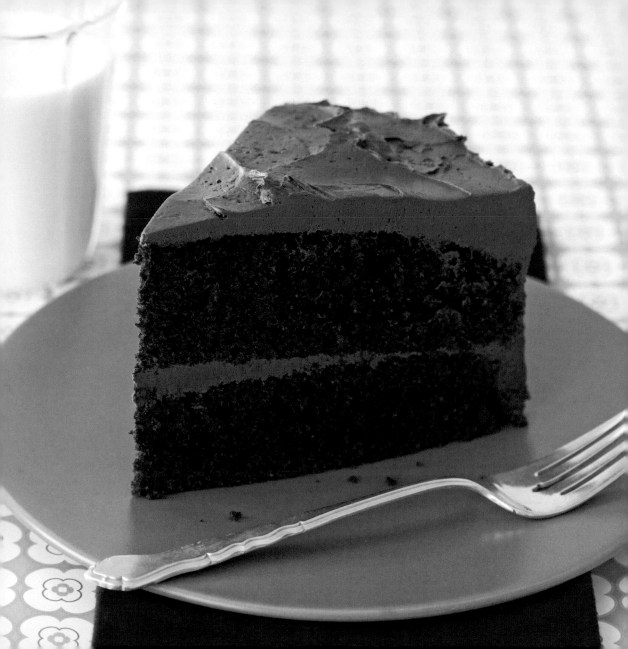

gift of the gods chocolate cake

This is my favorite fudge cake. It is light, but also buttery, chocolaty, soft, and moist. Its texture is strong enough to hold up to buttercream, which can drag a lesser cake down. This cake goes with each of the four icings presented in this chapter. **Makes 2 (8-inch) cake layers**

Preheat the oven to 350°F.

Prepare two standard cake pans (8 inches in diameter, 2 inches deep) by lightly spraying the bottoms and sides with cooking spray. Cut out circles of parchment paper to fit on the bottom of each pan. The paper should be flat, not inching up the sides of the pan. Set pans aside.

Mix together the cake flour, cocoa, baking soda, and salt in a bowl with a whisk and set aside.

Combine the chocolate, brown sugar, and milk in a stainless steel bowl and place over simmering water. Stir the ingredients together as they melt. This creates a chocolate base for the cake, which you can transfer to a big mixing bowl.

Put the butter in the bowl of an electric mixer fitted with the paddle attachment, and mix at medium speed until the butter is light and soft. Change to the whisk attachment, and slowly add the granulated sugar and continue whipping until light and fluffy. Add the egg yolks, one at a time, and beat until each one is incorporated. Add half of the dry ingredients and mix in slowly. Add half of the buttermilk. Repeat this process until all the flour mixture and milk is incorporated. This is your batter. Add the batter to the chocolate base and combine lightly using a large rubber spatula. Stir in the vanilla, then set aside. You now have a chocolate batter.

continued

Chocolate Choices

Barry Callebaut Origins (60% cacao or above), Lindt Dark, or Ghirardelli Premium

1³/₄ cups cake flour

1/4 cup unsweetened cocoa powder

1 teaspoon baking soda

1 teaspoon kosher salt

4 ounces dark chocolate, finely chopped

1 cup firmly packed light brown sugar

1/2 cup whole or 2% milk

1/2 cup (1 stick) cold unsalted butter

1/2 cup granulated sugar

3 large egg yolks

3/4 cup buttermilk

1 teaspoon vanilla extract

3 large egg whites

Thoroughly rinse and dry your mixer bowl and whisk attachment, then mix the egg whites at medium speed for about 3 minutes, or until they hold a medium peak. Gently fold half of the whipped egg whites into the chocolate batter until the mixture is smooth. Repeat with the remaining egg whites, and fold just until all the egg whites are incorporated. The egg whites should be fully incorporated—no streaks. Pour the completed cake batter into the prepared cake pans equally.

Bake for about 35 minutes, or until the cakes springs lightly in the center when touched, or a toothpick comes out clean with a few crumbs but no batter. Remove the cakes from the oven and cool on a rack until room temperature. Remove the cake layers by using a paring knife to gently cut the cake from the sides of the pan. Take a cake circle or sturdy paper plate, and place it over the pan. Invert the cake onto the plate and remove the parchment circle the cake baked on. Repeat this process for the other cake layer. Ice the first layer with the icing of your choice, with about 1/2 inch of icing on top. Place the second layer onto the cake with the bottom side up, which will give you a flat, undomed top. Ice the whole cake thinly (this is a crumb coat to stabilize the cake and hold the crumbs in place), chill it for at least 20 minutes, then apply a final coat of icing.

cocoa chantilly cream

The French named this dessert cream after a castle in the town of Chantilly, a culinary hot spot in the 1800s. If you love whipped cream and chocolate, you'll appreciate this long-lasting, perfect marriage. This recipe makes enough icing for 2 generous coats on a cake and decorations. **Makes 6 cups icing**

Sift together the cocoa powder, confectioners' sugar, and salt in small bowl and set aside.

Pour the cream and vanilla into the bowl of an electric mixer fitted with a wire whisk and whip for about 2 minutes at medium speed, or until the cream is visibly thick and will hold a medium peak. Stop the mixer, scoop up about 1/2 cup of the cream, and slowly add it to the bowl of cocoa and sugar. Whisk together until it forms a paste. Then add the paste back into the mixer bowl and whip until firm peaks form.

Chocolate Choices

Valrhona, Droste, or Scharffen Berger cocoa powder

1/2 cup unsweetened alkalized or dutched cocoa powder

1 1/4 cups confectioners' sugar

1/2 teaspoon salt

4 cups cold heavy cream

2 tablespoons vanilla extract

glaze of the gods

Here is a silky and easy-to-make chocolate glaze. It creates a thin layer of satiny chocolate for cakes, cupcakes, ice cream, and pound cake. The quality of the ingredients really counts in this one—use your best chocolate and butter! **Makes 2 cups glaze**

Chocolate Choices

Felchlin Cru Sauvage, Valrhona Manjari, or Lindt Creation 70% Pure Chocolate Bar

8 ounces dark chocolate, chopped

3/4 cup (1 1/2 sticks) unsalted butter, at room temperature

1 tablespoon light corn syrup

1 tablespoon Cognac

1 tablespoon vanilla extract

1/2 teaspoon kosher salt

Melt all the ingredients together in a stainless steel bowl over a saucepan with simmering water or over very low heat in a very heavy pot. Blend until the mixture is smooth and shiny. Pour over the prepared cake while the glaze is still warm. The excess glaze can be frozen and reheated for later use.

sugar islands chocolate buttercream

This recipe offers treasures of the Caribbean "sugar islands": chocolate, sugar, and rum. It's a classic French buttercream using a cooked sugar technique, *pâté à bombe*, to blend and aerate the eggs and sugar, which creates incomparable richness. Or maybe it's the butter. Or maybe it's the chocolate. You get the picture—it's rich! One batch makes enough to ice one 2-layer cake, but if you like generous layers and rosettes, double this recipe. Allow time to chill the buttercream. If soupy, chill it for another half hour. If stiff, heat it over a saucepan of hot water, then whip it. For children, you can omit the rum. Makes 3 1/2 cups icing

In the bowl of an electric mixer fitted with the whisk attachment, whip the egg yolks at medium speed for about a minute to add volume to them.

Meanwhile, in a small saucepan, stir together the sugar, corn syrup, and water. Remove any sugar crystals from the inner sides of the pan with a wet paper towel. Place the saucepan over medium heat and don't stir anymore. Allow the mixture to boil for 2 to 3 minutes, until it reaches the soft-ball stage, or 235°F on a digital (or candy) thermometer.

Stop the mixer, take off the wire whip and do the next step by hand. Carefully add a small splash of the hot sugar mixture into the egg yolks and briskly stir with the wire whisk. Once it is fully mixed, pour in a little more hot sugar and repeat . . . slowly . . . until all of the sugar mixture is incorporated into the yolks. Place the whip and the bowl back on the mixer and whip at medium speed for about 5 minutes, or until it becomes light and fluffy. Add pieces of butter, one at a time, while continuing to whip the buttercream. Stop the mixer and add the chocolate, vanilla, rum, cream, and salt. Allow the mixture to whip for another minute and taste your creation. Adjust the flavors, then chill and rewhip a little before using.

Chocolate Choices

Michel Cluizel Hacienda Los Anconès or Cacao Barry Origins Saint-Domingue

6 large egg yolks

3/4 cup sugar

2 tablespoons light corn syrup

1/4 cup water

1 1/4 cups (2 1/2 sticks) cold unsalted butter, cut into small pieces

12 ounces dark chocolate, melted

1 tablespoon vanilla extract

2 tablespoons dark rum, preferably Meyers's (optional)

Splash of heavy cream

1 teaspoon kosher salt

sweet bittersweet ganache

Ganache is one of the great creations of the chocolate world. It is a very versatile emulsion of melted chocolate and cream. It can be poured as a glaze, whipped to make icing, piped to decorate cakes, shaped into truffles, thickened with butter, flavored with alcohol and herbal infusions, or blended with fruit. While you can certainly make ganache by hand with warm chocolate, warm cream, and a whisk, the food-processor method, below, is favored by many pastry chefs and chocolatiers. The rapid action of the machine's blades creates a smooth texture and a very stable emulsion. Immersion blenders work well, too. If you envision a cake with thick icing layers and decorations, double this recipe. **Makes 2¹/₂ cups icing**

Chocolate Choices

Amadei dark and milk chocolate, or Scharffen Berger dark and milk chocolate

4 ounces milk chocolate, finely chopped

6 ounces dark chocolate, finely chopped

1 cup heavy cream

2 tablespoons light corn syrup

1 tablespoon honey

1 teaspoon vanilla extract

Put the dark and milk chocolates in a medium stainless steel bowl over a saucepan of simmering water and heat just until the chocolate melts, then transfer the warm chocolate to the bowl of a food processor. Meanwhile, heat the cream in a small saucepan over low heat just until it starts to simmer. Pour the warm cream into the warm chocolate and wait about 1 minute. Add the corn syrup, honey, and vanilla. Run the food processor. You'll notice that the mixture will look speckled and separated, then will come together as a uniform ganache. Adjust the flavors to taste.

black forest cupcakes

Take a tray of these to someone who deserves them—most kids love the look of them but prefer them without the alcohol. Just add a splash of vanilla instead of the Kirsch suggested below. If possible, buy ripe, tart black cherries (like Schmidt) in season. Otherwise, drained frozen or canned sour cherries will work, but avoid heavy syrups or cherry pie fillings. For tips on pitting fresh cherries, see page 59. If you want a shortcut, substitute 1 teaspoon vanilla extract for the vanilla bean. **Makes 16 iced cupcakes**

Preheat the oven to 350°F. Grease 16 muffin cups or line with baking cups.

Make the completed cake batter as directed. Ladle it into the prepared muffin pan, filling each cavity about three-quarters full. A big pastry bag works well for this job. Bake for about 25 minutes. The cupcake tops will form a dome and a toothpick inserted in the center should come out clean. Allow them to cool in the pan to room temperature.

While the cupcakes are baking, prepare the cherries. Combine the cherries, Kirsch, corn syrup, and salt in a small saucepan and heat over medium heat for 3 minutes. Then allow the mixture to cool.

Once the cupcakes have cooled, scoop out a big, round chunk of each top with a melon baller or a paring knife. This will later be filled in with Chantilly Cream and cherries.

To prepare the Chantilly Cream, sift the confectioners' sugar into a small bowl and set aside. Place the vanilla bean seeds in the bowl of an electric mixer fitted with the whisk attachment and let it run for several seconds at medium speed, which will release the flavor of the seeds.

continued

Cupcakes

Batter for Gift of the Gods Chocolate Cake (page 115)

Cherries

2 cups fresh, frozen, or canned sour cherries, pitted

3/4 cup Kirsch or brandy

1 tablespoon light corn syrup

1 teaspoon kosher or coarse salt

black forest cupcakes, *continued*

Chantilly Cream

1/2 cup confectioners' sugar

Seeds of 1 vanilla bean

2 cups heavy cream

Dark chocolate shavings,
for decoration

Stop the mixer, add the cream to the mixing bowl, and whip at medium speed for 1 to 2 minutes, until the cream reaches medium peaks. Stop the mixer, and mix several tablespoons of the cream into the bowl of confectioners' sugar to make a paste. Then add the sugar paste into the mixing bowl and continue whipping until stiff peaks form. You will see fluffy whipped cream speckled with black vanilla seeds.

To make the chocolate shavings, use a vegetable peeler or sharp chef's knife on a large block of room temperature dark chocolate and shave the chocolate into large curls. If only small pieces of chocolate are available, very finely chop them to make more of a chocolate dust. Set shavings/dust aside.

To assemble the cupcakes, take the scooped-out cupcakes out of their baking pan. Fill each one with a little whipped cream, then a generous scoop of drained, cooked cherries. Cover them up with another dollop of whipped cream, then chocolate shavings on top. Or try icing the entire cupcake with big whipped cream rosettes and adding a cherry on top along with the chocolate shavings. Indulgent!

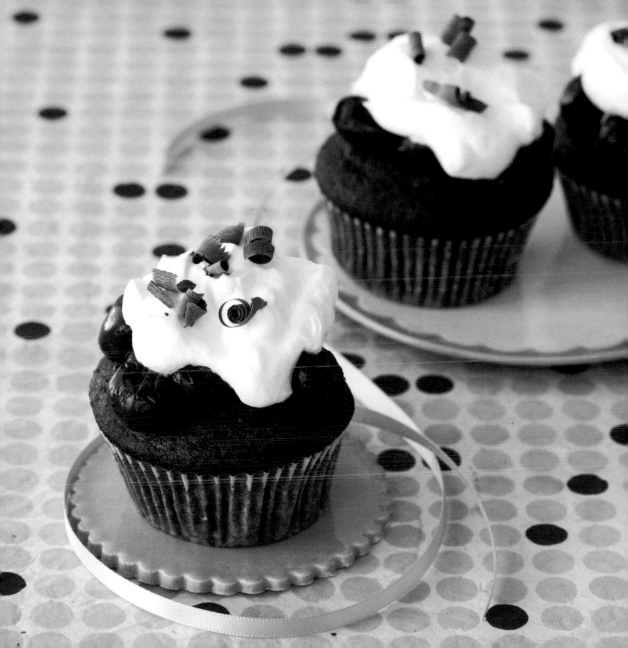

milk chocolate mousse muffins

Silicone baking pans bake evenly and won't rust after you wash them. They are pricey, but as a special gift for your friend or yourself, splurge! I buy a nice silicon muffin pan, use fancy baking cup liners, load them with this milk chocolate mousse, then wrap the pan up tightly with plastic wrap, tie it with a big bow, and freeze it. When you are ready to gift it, you'll give the satisfying sweetness of a softening mousse, the convenience of muffins, and a reusable piece of kitchenware. This is an all-purpose mousse that can also be served in a dish with cookies as a simple satisfying dessert. Note: Agar is a thickener available in health food stores. It is a substitute for gelatin and suitable for vegetarians. **Makes 12 muffins**

Chocolate Choices

E. Guittard dark and milk chocolate, or Amadei dark and milk chocolate

8 ounces dark chocolate, finely chopped

4 ounces milk chocolate, finely chopped

1 1/2 cups heavy cream

5 large egg yolks

1 whole large egg

1 tablespoon agar

1/4 cup sugar

2 tablespoons light corn syrup

3 tablespoons water

2 tablespoons bourbon or dark rum (optional)

1 tablespoon vanilla extract

Line a standard 12-cup muffin pan with baking cups.

Melt the two chocolates together in a stainless steel bowl over a pan of simmering water and set aside.

In the bowl of an electric mixer fitted with the whisk attachment, whip the cream for 3 to 5 minutes to form stiff peaks. Transfer the whipped cream to a bowl, cover with plastic wrap, and store in the refrigerator.

Rinse out the mixer bowl and the whisk attachment and return them to the mixer. Combine the egg yolks and whole egg in the bowl and mix on low until the eggs are frothy. Mix in the agar.

In a small saucepan, combine the sugar, corn syrup, and water. Bring to a full boil over medium heat. Boil for about 5 minutes, or until the mixture reaches 235°F on a candy or digital thermometer. Carefully add just a tiny splash of the hot syrup into the eggs, then turn the mixer on to low speed and beat for 1 minute. Add another small splash and beat for 30 seconds or so, then another, carefully and slowly incorporating all the hot sugar syrup into the eggs. Whip on medium speed for another 3 minutes.

Take the bowl off the mixer and gradually fold in the chocolate mixture with a big rubber spatula or wooden spoon. Once the mixture is smooth, gently fold in the whipped cream, bourbon, and vanilla. Blend gently until the mousse is smooth with no streaks.

Using a big pastry bag with a big star tip, pipe the mousse into the baking cups until they look like big ice cream cones. Chill until you are ready to serve or freeze them, then wrap them up to present as a gift.

bliss byte: chef's quote

It is not so easy to make chocolate. Sometimes, we have to balance the crazy beans.

—Chef Jacques Torres, Chocolate Haven, New York

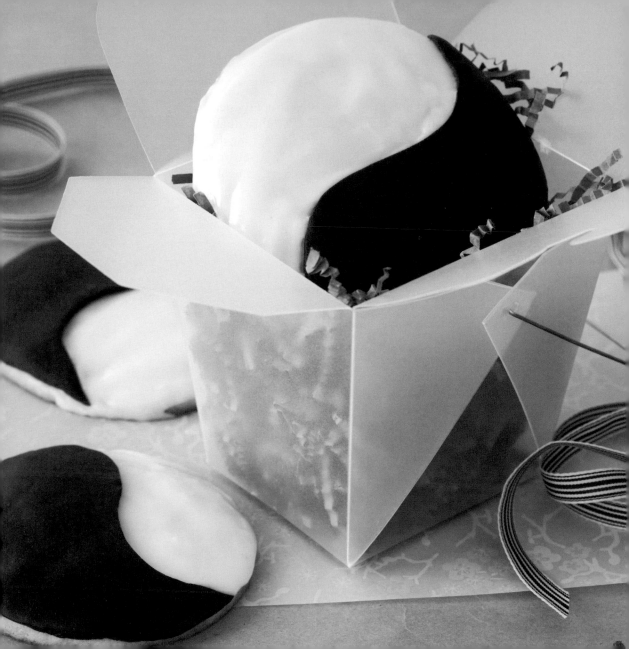

yin yang cookies

These playful black-and-white cookies have the simple appeal of chocolate and vanilla as well as the universally appealing symbol of Buddhist duality, yin and yang. By giving these cookies as a gift, you get the return gift of delighting the recipient. For the shortening, look for an all-natural transfat-free brand, available in many health food stores. Use Dark Chocolate Plastique (page 134) to make the chocolate side of the yin yang decoration. **Makes 25 to 30 cookies**

Sift together the flour, salt, and baking soda and set aside.

In an electric mixer fitted with the paddle attachment, beat the butter at low speed for a minute or two until soft. Add the shortening and sugar and continue beating until fluffy. Add the eggs, vanilla, corn syrup, and almond extract and increase the speed to medium for about 1 minute. Stop the mixer and add half of the flour mixture, then beat slowly until all the flour is incorporated. Next, add half the sour cream, then mix slowly. Repeat until all the flour mixture and sour cream are incorporated. Allow the dough to rest in the refrigerator for about 20 minutes.

While the dough chills, make the icing. Sift the confectioners' sugar into a bowl. Combine the corn syrup and water in a saucepan over medium heat and bring to a boil. Stir the hot mixture into the confectioners' sugar, stirring vigorously. Add the butter and vanilla and stir until the mixture is smooth. Transfer the mixture to a bowl and store at room temperature until the cookies are ready to be iced.

Preheat the oven to 350°F.

Scoop a ball of cookie dough (about 1/4 cup) onto the cookie sheet one at a time, placing them about 1 inch

continued

Cookies

3 cups all purpose flour

1 teaspoon kosher salt

1/4 teaspoon baking soda

3/4 cups (11/2 sticks) cold unsalted butter

1/2 cup shortening

11/2 cups sugar

2 large eggs

1 tablespoon vanilla extract

1 tablespoon light corn syrup

1/2 teaspoon almond extract or Cognac

1/3 cup sour cream

Icing

3 cups confectioners' sugar

1/4 cup light corn syrup

3 tablespoons unsalted butter, melted

1 teaspoon vanilla extract

3 tablespoons water

Decoration

1 pound Dark Chocolate Plastique (page 134)

apart. Roll each cookie scoop into a ball between your palms and flatten each one slightly to a thickness of at least 1/2 inch.

Bake the cookies for 10 minutes, or until slightly risen and golden brown on the edges.

Remove them from the baking sheet with a spatula, and place them on a plate. Ice the cookies by spreading a thin layer of icing on each one with an offset spatula while they are still warm.

To decorate, make a batch or 1/2 batch of Dark Chocolate Plastique (the recipe yields more than you will need here but freezes well). I like using a round pastry tip and a paring knife to cut out shapes. Roll out the plastique on parchment paper until very thin. Cut a yin yang shape (like a large comma) with a paring knife to fit on the top of your cookie. Use an offset spatula to move the plastique comma onto the iced cookie. You need only one side, because when you place the plastique on the iced cookie, it will stick, creating the black-and-white, yin yang pattern. This may involve some trial and error to get just the right fit, but it becomes easy as you go along. You can use your pastry tip to punch out the "eye" of the yin yang symbol before you place it on the cookie for the full effect.

earthquake cookies in a jar

These cookies are familiarly fudgey like a good brownie, cute because of the crinkles or "faults" that cut through their warm sugary surfaces, and they travel well to picnics or friends' houses. Pile them up in a mason jar and tie them with a bow. **Makes about 40 cookies**

Sift together the flour, baking powder, almond meal, and salt. Melt the chocolate and butter together in a stainless steel bowl over a pan of simmering water.

In an electric mixer fitted with a whisk, whip together the eggs and sugar at high speed for 3 to 4 minutes, until they become fluffy. Add the melted chocolate mixture and mix until incorporated. Add the dry ingredients slowly (better to take your bowl off the mixer for this part so flour doesn't fly around your kitchen) and mix until incorporated. Stir in the coffee, vanilla, and rum. Transfer to a small bowl and refrigerate for about an hour. It will become firm.

Preheat the oven to 350°F. Line a cookie sheet with parchment paper. Put the granulated sugar in one bowl and the confectioners' sugar in a second bowl.

Using a sturdy spoon, scoop the chilled dough into 1-inch scoops and place them 1 inch apart on the prepared cookie sheet. Roll each individual cookie between your hands until it is a smooth ball, dip in the bowl of granulated sugar, then in the bowl of confectioners' sugar, coating each one fully. Return them to the cookie sheet.

Bake for about 10 minutes, or until the sugar cracks and the cookies just start to firm up. (They are especially delicious with a little softness in the center.) Allow them to cool on a rack, then store airtight.

1/2 cup all-purpose flour

3/4 teaspoon baking powder

1 cup almond meal (also known as ground almonds)

1 teaspoon kosher salt

12 ounces dark chocolate, finely chopped

1/4 cup (1/2 stick) unsalted butter, at room temperature

3 large eggs

1/2 cup sugar

3 tablespoons brewed coffee

2 tablespoons vanilla extract

1 tablespoon rum

Decorating Sugar

3/4 cup granulated sugar

3/4 cup sifted confectioners' sugar

white chocolate roses

Doughlike chocolate, often called *chocolate plastique*, makes cake decorations that are as beautiful to eat as they are to admire. The simple technique is the same for Dark Chocolate Plastique (page 134), but here the delicate ivory color allows you more opportunities for creating realistic, elegant flowers suitable for weddings and gifts. For a gift, I like to present the roses in a reusable box, such as a small jewelry box lined with plastic wrap, with the white chocolate roses inside. Import shops often sell ethnic boxes and are a great place to pick these up. Or, gently place the roses into a flower vase packed with truffles or cookies. **Makes about 25 roses**

1 1/2 pounds White Chocolate Plastique (page 135)

Food color

Soften the white chocolate plastique so that it is malleable. Knead the mixture on parchment paper as if it were bread dough. It should feel dry to the touch like Play-Doh, and you should be able to mold small chunks of it without it sticking to your fingers. If it is too sticky, you can sift some cornstarch over it to dry it up. Divide the dough into 3 or 4 different disks if you plan to knead in food coloring. To color the plastique, use parchment paper over your work surface and latex or vinyl gloves. Add a few drops of food color to each disk of white chocolate plastique to create different hues for roses and leaves. Knead the color in until it is fully incorporated and you achieve the shade you like.

For the roses, roll out a disk of the plastique on parchment paper with a rolling pin as if it were a pie dough. Roll it until it is thin, about 1/4 inch. Then, make small circles using the back of a pastry bag tip. If you don't have a pastry bag tip, you can use a bottle top from a milk jug or anything that will cut uniform circles about 1 inch in diameter. Separate the circles (which we will now call "petals") on the parchment paper, and flatten the outer edges of each petal with the back of a spoon to make them almost transparent.

Peel up the first petal off the parchment paper (a small offset spatula helps with this job) and roll it tight, like a cigar. Pick up the next petal and wrap it around the first one. Each petal should get successively looser and wider, mimicking the way a rose in full bloom opens. You can attach as many petals as you like to create the style of rose bouquet you want. Place each completed rose on a plate covered with parchment paper, wrap the plate with plastic wrap, and put in the refrigerator until you are ready to use them.

To make leaves to round out your bouquet, add a few drops of green food coloring to a disk of the white chocolate plastique, roll it out thinly as above, then use a paring knife to cut free-form leaf shapes. Once you have completed a number of roses and leaves, you can form a bouquet in a plastic cup that fits inside a flower vase.

chocolate in the arts: painting

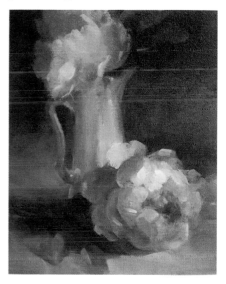

Tarzier's *Peonies and Chocolate Pot*.

Reprinted by permission of Carol Tarzier, www.tarzier.com

appendix I: mix and match basic recipes

These mix and match basics can be used as building blocks for cakes and desserts and will become classics in your baking repertoire.

chocolate sugar dough

This recipe works for chocolate tart crusts, chocolate sugar cookies, and as a cheesecake base. You can keep a batch in the freezer to be ready for any dessert challenge that arises. Although the method given below is safer in terms of overmixing, if you are in a rush, toss all the ingredients in a food processor and pulse a few times until you get a smooth dough. **Makes about 2 pounds dough**

1 1/2 cups sifted cake flour

3/4 cup unsweetened cocoa powder

1/2 teaspoon kosher salt

3/4 cup (1 1/2 sticks) cold unsalted butter

1 cup sugar

1 large egg

1 tablespoon rum

1 tablespoon brewed espresso or coffee

1 teaspoon vanilla extract

Sift together the cake flour, cocoa powder, and salt into a medium bowl, and stir with a whisk. Set aside.

In the bowl of an electric mixer fitted with the paddle attachment, cream the butter at low speed for about 2 minutes, or until it is soft and fluffy. Slowly beat in the sugar. Add the egg and mix on low. Turn off the mixer and slowly add half of the dry ingredients, and continue mixing on low until incorporated. Add the other half, then the rum, coffee, and vanilla and mix until smooth.

Remove the dough and form it into a disk, then cover it with plastic wrap or put it in a sealable plastic bag. Chill it for at least 30 minutes.

With a rolling pin, flatten the dough between two layers of parchment paper. Sprinkle the dough with a little flour if it is sticking to the parchment paper. Roll it into a disk about 1/2 inch thick and store in the refrigerator until ready to use.

vanilla sugar dough

This classic sugar cookie and tart shell dough is also known as *pâte sucrée*. Like the Chocolate Sugar Dough, it is very versatile and works as tart shells or sugar cookies, or whenever you need a sweet, sturdy crust to hold delicacies like strawberries and cream or chocolate mousse. You can also mix all the ingredients in a food processor—just pulse until the ingredients come together. **Makes about 2 pounds dough**

Cream the butter in the bowl of an electric mixer fitted with the paddle attachment at low speed until it is soft. Switch to the whisk attachment and slowly add the sugar while continuing to beat. Add the egg yolks, cream, vanilla, and salt and mix on low until smooth. Stop the mixer and add half of the flour. Mix on low until smooth, then add the rest of the flour. Mix until smooth. Remove from the mixer bowl, flatten the dough into a disk, wrap in plastic wrap, and chill for at least 30 minutes until ready to use.

1 cup (2 sticks) cold unsalted butter

1/2 cup sugar

2 large egg yolks

2 tablespoons heavy cream

1 tablespoon vanilla extract

1 teaspoon kosher salt

2 1/2 cups flour, sifted

bliss byte: chef's quote

Vanilla is the salt and pepper of the bakeshop. We use it in everything.

—Chef Norma Salazar, California School of Culinary Arts

dark chocolate plastique

This is a miracle of culinary chemistry. This simple mix of melted chocolate and corn syrup renders the chocolate pliable enough to shape, yet firm enough to hold its form once you craft it. Makes chocolate flowers, letters, animals—any decoration you can dream up. **Makes 1 1/2 pounds plastique**

16 ounces chocolate, finely chopped (2 cups)

1 cup light corn syrup

Melt the chocolate in a stainless steel bowl over a pan of simmering water. Once the chocolate is melted, stir in the corn syrup. Remove from the heat and allow the mixture to come to room temperature, stirring occasionally. The chocolate plastique should come together with the consistency of a pie dough or a slightly melted Tootsie Roll, and it will become more flexible as you work with it. Roll it out on a work surface covered with parchment paper. Roll it thin (about 1/4 inch) in order to cut designs with cookie cutters. Store the remaining chocolate plastique covered at room temperature or in the freezer in a tightly wrapped sealable plastic freezer bag.

great books on chocolate artistry

The Art of Chocolate by Elaine Gonzalez. A bilingual expert on chocolate history makes chocolate sculptures that inspire home cooks.

Chocolate: Behind the Scenes by Philippe Bertrand and Philippe Marand. Chocolate artists teach you how to make chocolate sculptures.

Discover Chocolate by Clay Gordon. Detailed and technical information about making, tasting, and evaluating chocolate. The author also moderates TheChocolateLife.com.

white chocolate plastique

This white chocolate plastique makes the perfect modeling chocolate, and the ivory color is beautiful on its own or can easily be combined with food coloring for colored flowers, leaves, and holiday decorations. It works very much like the dark chocolate version (opposite page), but it needs a smaller amount of corn syrup and a little cornstarch.
Makes 1 1/2 pounds plastique

Melt the chocolate over in a stainless steel bowl over a saucepan of simmering water, and stir in the corn syrup, then the cornstarch. Allow the mixture to come to room temperature, stirring occasionally. If your room is warm, put the plastique in the refrigerator for 10 minutes or so for it to firm up. If you plan to add food coloring to part of the batch, this is the right time to knead it in. It should come together with the consistency of a pie dough or a slightly melted Tootsie Roll, and it will become more flexible as you work with it. Store the plastique wrapped in plastic or in a sealable plastic bag.

16 ounces white chocolate, finely chopped
3/4 cup light corn syrup
1/4 cup cornstarch, sifted

simple secret icing

Here's the simple secret to winning a chocolate lover's heart: we want chocolate, butter, and sugar . . . and make it fluffy, please. **Makes 3 cups icing**

4 ounces milk chocolate, finely chopped

1 cup (2 sticks) unsalted cold butter, plus more as needed for thickness

1 cup confectioners' sugar, sifted

1/4 cup unsweetened cocoa powder

1/4 cup boiling water

3 tablespoons heavy cream, plus more as needed

2 tablespoons vanilla extract

1 teaspoon kosher salt

Melt the chocolate in a stainless steel bowl over a pan of simmering water or in a warm oven and set aside.

Cream the butter in the bowl of an electric mixer fitted with the paddle attachment at medium speed until very soft. Switch to the whisk attachment, add the confectioners' sugar, and continue whipping at medium speed for a minute or two, stopping the mixer to scrape the bottom and sides of the bowl as needed. This mixture should be very soft and fluffy.

Combine the cocoa powder and water in a mixing cup or small bowl and stir it into a warm paste. Allow it to cool a little. This is your cocoa paste.

Add the melted milk chocolate, cocoa paste, cream, vanilla, and salt to the mixing bowl and whip at low speed until smooth. If it is too thin to spread onto a cake or cookie and hold its shape, chill it for 20 minutes or so. If it is still too thin, whisk in some more butter and chill again. If it is too thick, add a little more cream. Chill the icing with the whip attachment in the bowl; whip it up one last time before using.

appendix II: shopping sources guide

Love chocolate? Love to shop? They go together like you and your best friend on an afternoon of January sales. This is my personal list of outstanding chocolate suppliers.

bakeware and tools

Chocolate Molds. Tomric Systems (www.tomric.com) has the best selection of chocolate molds in the country. JB Prince (www.jbprince.com) provides top-of-the-line molds and pans.

General Equipment. Chef Rubber (www.chefrubber.com) features colored cocoa butter, silicone molds, spatulas, power tools, and gadgetry. Kerekes (www.bakedeco.com) offers chocolate transfer sheets, bowls, cake pans, spatulas, gadgets, and decorating materials geared toward the professional with reasonable prices.

Offset Spatulas. Any kitchen store will have them in either full size or small—both are great for chocolate work and cake decorating. Three online sources are Sur La Table (www.surlatable.com), Surfas (www.surfasonline.com), and Bed Bath and Beyond (www.bedbathandbeyond.com).

Tempering Machines. These are for the serious candy maker interested in molding and dipping bonbons. My favorite is American Chocolate Mould Company's Table Top Temperer (www.americanchocolatemould.com). Another popular source for machines for home use is Chocovision (www.chocovision.com).

Thermometers. Digital thermometers really help with tempering. Most kitchen stores have them, or you can order one from Taylor (www.taylorusa.com). My favorites are the all-purpose Weekend Warrior and the oven thermometer.

chocolate, chocolate, chocolate

Here are some of my top favorite couvertures. Most are available through www.chocosphere .com or directly from the companies as indicated in the list that follows.

Amedei. www.amedei.com. Powerful yet sweet flavors from an Italian chocolate company steeped in the Swiss tradition. Their Milk Chocolate Bar 32% is especially smooth and rich.

Barry Callebaut. www.barry-callebaut.com. This company leads the industry in supporting sustainable farming, organic chocolate, and ethical production, and their Origins line (from their Cacao Barry brand) offers a range of carefully crafted flavors.

Chocolates El Rey. www.elreychocolate.com. Search the world and you'll be challenged to find a better white chocolate. El Rey, located in Venezuela's legendary growing region, also produces a selection of excellent darks.

Domori. www.domorichocolate.com. This Italian brand appeals to chocolate lovers with a taste for complex darks.

Felchlin. www.felchlin.com. This Swiss company prides itself on its bean selection, with offerings such as "Cru Sauvage" made from wild cacao trees in Venezuela.

Guittard Chocolate Company. www.eguittard.com. Long a supplier for California's favorite candy shops, this company now produces excellent, high-quality couvertures under the brand name E. Guittard. Try the Quetzalcoatl 72% Cacao Mass Bittersweet bar.

Lindt and Sprüngli. www.lindt.com. Bars of Lindt couverture are easy to find in quality grocery stores in the United States. Sprüngli is the name of a brilliant group of confectionary shops in Zurich (see page 141).

Michel Cluizel. www.chocolatmichelcluizel-na.com. Prized by the Europeans as elegant and masterfully made, Michel Cluizel is available in specialty shops.

Omanhene. www.omanhene.com. Unlike most chocolate companies, this one is based in the growing region of Ghana in Africa, and features dark chocolate with smoothness and power.

Pralus. www.chocolats-pralus.com. Smooth, sophisticated, chic—everything you might expect from a top French chocolate company.

Scharffen Berger Chocolate Maker. www.scharffenberger.com. This pioneering California brand is now owned by Hershey's; production of its premium couvertures will continue in Illinois and the flavor will live on. Strong darks, nuanced milks, and top-notch natural cocoa powder and nibs.

Trader Joe's. www.traderjoes.com. Trader Joe's Pound Plus 72% is a sharp Belgian couverture in big volume for a very good price. Available in Trader Joe's stores, not online.

Valrhona. www.valrhona.com. This company is widely considered the best chocolate maker in the world. Great craftsmanship, expertise, bean selection, refined taste, and attention to detail. My favorites are Jivara Lactée, Manjari, and cocoa powder.

top artisan chocolatiers in the united states

Artisan chocolatiers work in small shops. They are usually not franchised, but most have online shops and will ship across the country (and sometimes across the world) happily. Here's where you get your bonbons!

Burdick Chocolates, Walpole, New Hampshire. www.burdickchocolate.com. The couverture is fragrant, the handmade designs (little chocolate mice) are unique. Burdick has a restaurant and chocolate school in New Hampshire and a chocolate café in Cambridge, Massachusetts.

Chocolate Haven, New York, New York. www.chocolatehaven.com. Celebrity chocolatier Jacques Torres works in open factories and offers bean-to-bar chocolates in every imaginable flavor.

Chocolate Springs Café, Lenox, Massachusetts. www.chocolatesprings.com. A wellspring of quality bonbons, glorious cakes, ice cream, bath products, and a chocolate reading room make this an inviting cocoa-café.

Chocopologie Café, Norwalk, Connecticut. www.knipschildt.com. Founded by award-winning chocolatier Fritz Knipschildt, this café offers beautiful bonbons and a window into the confection-making process.

Garrison Confections, Providence, Rhode Island. www.garrsionconfections.com. Seasonal flavors and colorful chocolate squares showcase this chocolatier's originality and skill.

Harbor Sweets, Salem, Massachusetts. www.harborsweets.com. A white chocolate toffee sailboat is the charming signature confection of this old-fashioned chocolatier.

Jade Chocolatier, San Francisco, California. www.jadechocolate.com. This online boutique offers chocolate infused with exotic tropical flavors.

Jin Patisserie, Venice, California. www.jinpatisserie.com. Quiet delicacy in design and brightness of flavor are the hallmarks.

Kees Chocolates, New York, New York. www.keeschocolates.com. Asian flavor infusions and fresh ingredients distinguish this small SoHo shop.

Lake Champlain Chocolates, Burlington, Vermont. www.lakechamplainchocolates.com. Traditional candy making and organic sensibilities harmonize in this picturesque chocolate factory.

Lillie Belle Farms, Central Point, Oregon. www.lilliebellefarms.com. Organic fruits grown by the farmer/chocolatier of this farmstand chocolate shop create an authentic product mix.

Marie Belle, New York, New York. www.mariebelle.com. Artists create fanciful chocolates topped with brightly colored purses, geometric designs, and more.

Moonstruck Chocolatier, Portland, Oregon. www.moonstruckchocolates.com. This chocolate company, featuring old-fashioned sweetness and handmade techniques, has five locations in Oregon.

Norman Love Confections, Fort Meyers, Florida. www.normanloveconfections.com. This celebrated confectioner leads the pack in hand-painted colored designs that pique the curiosity.

Recchiuti Confections, San Francisco, California. www.recchiuticonfections.com. Innovation and creativity make this award-winning shop consistently excellent. Burnt caramel, Kona coffee, tea-flavored chocolates, s'mores, and sauces are house specialties.

Valerie Confections, Los Angeles, California. www.valerieconfections.com. Sleek black squares of dark chocolate encase perfectly amber toffee in this shop's signature confection.

Vosges Haut-Chocolat, Chicago, Illinois. www.vosgeschocolate.com. Truffles infused with flavors from around the world are center stage in this stylish chocolate shop with locations in Chicago, New York, and Las Vegas.

top international artisan chocolatiers

Bernachon, Paris. www.bernachon.com. Famed chocolatier takes chocolate from bean to bar in the Old World tradition.

La Maison du Chocolat, Paris. www.lamaisonduchocolat.com. This powerhouse of artisan chocolates was founded by Robert Linxe, who uses the best chocolate traditions with both classic and daring flavors.

Lenôtre, Paris. www.lenotre.com. Dynamic Parisian pastry chef Gaston Lenôtre created this empire of pastry arts, which includes shops worldwide and culinary schools.

Lindt & Sprüngli, Zurich. www.sprungli.com. The storied Swiss confectionary shop, Sprüngli, merged with Lindt to form a company with something for everyone. While Lindt's website sells familiar Easter bunnies and bars, Sprüngli's sites sell exquisite handmade confections. Their English language website links to their Dubai shop (their main site is in German).

Mary Chocolates, Brussels and Tokyo. www.marychoc.com; www.mary.co.jp. This shop features superlative Belgian designs, and the Tokyo shop specializes in uniquely beautiful Asian flavors and floral, hand-piped chocolate artworks.

Neuhaus, Brussels. www.neuhaus.online-store.com. Credited with inventing the filled, bite-size chocolate confection (now known as a "praline" or "bonbon") and the ballotine box in which to present them, Neuhaus has a long history as one of Belgium's finest.

Peter Marcolini, Paris. www.marcolini.be. "Haute Couture of Chocolate" is the approach Peter Marcolini takes to his many upscale boutiques around the world.

Pierre Hermé, Paris. www.pierreherme.com. Called "the Picasso of pastry" by *Vogue* magazine, Pierre Hermé runs deluxe pastry chocolate shops in Paris and Tokyo.

Richart, Paris and New York. www.richart-chocolates.com. Irresistible squares of dark chocolates encasing vibrant flavors make this chocolatier a favorite.

Thomas Haas Fine Chocolates, Vancouver. www.thomashaas.com. Thomas Haas, trained in both the European confectionary tradition and fine dining, offers sophisticated squares and bonbons.

Wittamer, Brussels. www.wittamer.com. This classic Belgian chocolate company combines fine ingredients, artistry, and freshness.

other ingredients

Cocoa Butter. Cocoa butter is useful in chocolate work, skin care products, and extra-rich fillings and icings. It can also can be colored and used to paint bonbons. Chocolate suppliers, such as www.chocolatesource.com and www.qzina.com, are good sources for 100% pure cocoa butter. Also, try www.cocoasupply.com. For colored cocoa butter, go to www.chefrubber.com.

Cocoa Powder and Nibs. Organic Nectar (www.organicnectars.com) makes minimally processed cocoa powder and cocoa nibs to preserve antioxidant power. You can also try Scharffen Berger (www.scharffenberger.com).

Edible Gold Decorations. Available at The Gold Leaf Company (www.goldleafcompany.com) or Chef Rubber (www.chefrubber.com).

Natural Food Colors. With natural decorating colors from India Tree in Seattle, Washington (www.indiatree.com), you can add a boost of color to icings without worrying about chemicals.

Packaging Materials. Have some fun when presenting candies and baked goods as gifts. King Arthur Flour (www.kingarthurflour.com) has a good selection. Thinking of starting a candy business? Nashville Wraps has great wholesale selections (www.nashvillewraps.com).

Ribbon Coconut. Also known as unsweetened coconut flakes, the coconut pieces are bigger and less sweet than the shredded version and can be lightly toasted for a dramatic decorative effect. Try Bakers C&C (www.bakerscandc.web-ctr.net).

Transfer Sheets. Chocolatiers create colorful, uniform designs of tinted cocoa butter that can be transferred onto bonbons or desserts. American Chocolate Designs (www.AmericanChocolate Designs.com) will make artistic custom cocoa butter transfer sheets for you; you can also try www.chefrubber.com or www.cheaptransfersheets.com.

Vanilla Beans and Extracts. Vanilla specialists Nielsen-Massey (www.nielsenmassey.com) make a delightful chocolate extract in addition to their wide selection of vanilla beans and vanilla extracts. Other sources for vanilla beans include the Boston Vanilla Bean Company (www.bostonvanillabeans.com), and the Vanilla Company (www.vanilla.com).

skin care

Chocolate Lotion. The Chocolate Mousse Hydration Masque from Eminence Organic Skin Care (www.eminenceorganics.com) smells like chocolate mousse because it is made with pure cocoa.

Cinnamon Cocoa Soap. Pacifica Mexican Cocoa Natural Soap contains spicy cinnamon and cocoa in a dark bar. It is available at Whole Foods or www.pacificasoaps.com.

Cocoa Butter Lotion. Palmer's Cocoa Butter Products offers a good cocoa butter lotion at www.etbrowne.com. For an unscented lotion base, try Michaels crafts store (www.michaels.com).

Orange Chocolate Soap. Orange Chocolate Soap from Fresh (www.fresh.com) smells fruity and perfumed instead of soapy. Fresh also carries fragrances with chocolate notes.

Peppermint Lotion. Peppermint Cooling Foot Lotion from the Body Shop (www.thebodyshop.com) is perfect for blending with a little melted chocolate.

Unscented Lotions. The After Bath Fresh Unscented Moisturizer from Epicuren (www.epicuren.com) is a luxurious unscented lotion that allows you to add cocoa extract or fragrance to your heart's content. On a budget? Try Eucerin, an unscented lotion from your local drug store (or www.eucerinus.com).

Unscented Soap. Unscented soap base can be found at Michaels crafts store (www.michaels.com).

publications

Dessert Professional. www.dessertprofessional.com. A magazine devoted to the pastry arts, including chocolate production, plated desserts, and ice cream.

Cocoaroma. www.cocoaroma.com. Brilliant photographs make you want to jump into this magazine, which explores chocolate's growing regions and celebrates its artisan chocolatiers.

bibliography

Almond, Steve. *Candy Freak*. New York: Algonquin, 2004.

Ayral, Dominique. *A Passion for Chocolate*. London, UK: Cassell, 2001.

Bailleux, Nathalie, Herve Bizeul, John Feltwell, Regine Kopp, Corby Kummer, Pierre Labanne, Cristina Pauly, Odile Perrard, and Mariarosa Schiaffino. *The Book of Chocolate*. Paris: Flammarion, 1995.

Beckett, Stephen T. *The Science of Chocolate*. Royal Society of Chemistry, Cambridge, UK, 2000.

Beranbaum, Rose Levy, and Maurice and Jean-Jacques Bernachon. *A Passion for Chocolate*. New York: Morrow, 1989.

Bergin, Mary, and Judy Gethers. *Spago Chocolate*. New York: Random House, 1999.

Bertrand, Philippe, and Philippe Marand. *Chocolate: Behind the Scenes*. France: Kirra Edition, 2003.

Bloom, Carole. *All About Chocolate*. New York: Macmillan, 1998.

Bowden, Jonny. *The 150 Healthiest Foods on Earth*. Gloucester, MA: Fair Winds Press, 2007.

Boyle, Tish, and Tim Moriarty. *Chocolate Passion: Recipes and Inspiration from the Kitchens of Chocolatier Magazine*. Hoboken, NJ: Wiley, 1999.

Brenner, Joel Glenn. *The Emperors of Chocolate: Inside the Secret World of Hershey and Mars*. New York: Broadway Books, 2000.

Brillat-Savarin, Jean-Anthelme. *The Physiology of Taste*. London: Penguin, 1970.

Coady, Chantal. *Real Chocolate: Sweet and Savory Recipes for Nature's Purest Form of Bliss*. London: Quadrille, 2003.

———. *The Chocolate Companion*. New York: Simon & Schuster, 1995.

Coe, Michael D. *Breaking the Maya Code*. New York: Thames & Hudson, 1996.

Coe, Sophie D. *America's First Cuisines*. Austin, TX: University of Texas Press, 1994.

Coe, Sophie D., and Michael D. Coe. *The True History of Chocolate*. London: Thames & Hudson, 1996.

Corriher, Shirley O. *Bakewise: The How and Whys of Successful Baking*. New York: Scribner, 2008.

Davidson, Alan. *The Oxford Companion to Food*. Oxford, UK: Oxford University Press, 1999.

Desaulniers, Marcel. *Death by Chocolate*. New York: Kenan Books, 1992.

Doutre-Roussel, Chloe. *The Chocolate Connoisseur: For Everyone with a Passion for Chocolate*. New York: Jeremy B. Tarcher/Penguin Group, 2005.

Drummond, Karen Eich, and Lisa M. Brefere. *Nutrition for Foodservice and Culinary Professionals*. Hoboken, NJ: Wiley, 2004.

Duchene, Laurent and Bridge Jones. *Le Cordon Bleu Dessert Techniques*. London: Carroll and Brown, 1999.

Escoffier, Auguste. *Le Guide Culinaire*. New York: Van Nostrand Reinhold, 1979.

Figoni, Paula. *How Baking Works: Exploring the Fundamentals of Baking Science*. Hoboken, NJ: Wiley, 2004.

Friberg, Bo. *The Advanced Professional Pastry Chef*. Hoboken, NJ: Wiley, 2003.

———. *The Professional Pastry Chef*. Hoboken, NJ: Wiley, 2002.

Gisslen, Wayne. *Professional Baking*. New York: Wiley, 2001.

Glassner, Barry. *The Gospel of Food*. New York: Ecco/Harper Collins, 2007.

———. *The Culture of Fear*. New York: Basic Books, 2000.

Gonzalez, Elaine. *The Art of Chocolate: Techniques and Recipes for Simply Spectacular Desserts and Confections*. New York: Chronicle Books, 1998.

Gordon, Clay. *Discover Chocolate*. New York: Gotham, 2007.

Greweling, Peter P. *Chocolate & Confections: Formula, Theory, and Technique for the Artisan Confectioner*. Hoboken, NJ: Wiley with The Culinary Institute of America, 2007.

Grivetti, Louis E. *Chocolate: History, Culture, and Heritage*. New York: Wiley, 2009.

Grun, Bernard. *The Timetables of History*. New York: Simon & Schuster, 1991.

Heatter, Maida. *Maida Heatter's Book of Great Chocolate Desserts*. New York: Knopf, 1978.

Jacobsen, Rowan. *Chocolate Unwrapped: The Surprising Health Benefits of America's Favorite Passion*. Montpelier, VT: Invisible Cities Press, 2003.

Jones, Prudence, and Nigel Pennick. *A History of Pagan Europe*. London: Routledge, 1995.

Kimmerle, Beth. *Chocolate: The Sweet History*. Portland, OR: Collector's Press, 2005.

Knight, Ian. *Chocolate and Cocoa. Health and Nutrition*. Oxford, UK: Blackwell Science, 1999.

Lebovitz, David. *The Great Book of Chocolate*. Berkeley, CA: Ten Speed Press, 2004.

Lopez, Ruth. *Chocolate: The Nature of Indulgence*. New York: Harry N. Abrams, 2002.

Malgieri, Nick. *Chocolate: From Simple Cookies to Extravagant Showstoppers*. New York: Morrow, 1998.

McGee, Harold. *On Food and Cooking: The Science and Lore of the Kitchen*. New York: Scribner, 1984.

Medrich, Alice. *Bittersweet*. New York: Artisan, 2003.

Mercier, Jacques. *The Temptation of Chocolate*. Paris: Lannoo, 2008.

Minifie, Bernard W. *Chocolate, Cocoa and Confectionery*. New Delhi, India: CBS Publishers & Distributors, 1989.

Montagné, Prosper. *La Rousse Gastronomique*. Edited by Jean-Francois Revel. New York: Clarkson Potter, 2001.

Morton, Marcia, and Frederic Morton. *Chocolate: An Illustrated History*. New York: Random House Value Publishing, 2006.

Off, Carol. *Bitter Chocolate*. New York: The New Press, 2006.

Pollan, Michael. *An Omnivore's Dilemma*. New York: Penguin, 2007.

———. *In Defense of Food*. New York: Penguin, 2008.

Presilla, Maricel E. *The New Taste of Chocolate*. Berkeley, CA: Ten Speed Press, 2009.

Rain, Patricia. *Vanilla: The Cultural History of the World's Favorite Flavor and Fragrance*. New York: Jeremy P. Tarcher/Penguin, 2004.

Rombauer, Irma S., and Marion Rombauer Becker. *The Joy of Cooking*. New York: Plume, 1997.

Rosenblum, Mort. *Chocolate: A Bittersweet Saga of Dark and Light*. New York: North Point Press, 2005.

Rykiel, Sonia, and Irene Frain. *Le Guide du Club des Croqueurs de Chocolat*. Neuilly-sur-Seine, France: Michel Lafon, 2003.

Scharffenberger, John, and Robert Steinberg. *The Essence of Chocolate: Recipes for Baking and Cooking with Fine Chocolate*. New York: Hyperion, 2006.

Schlosser, Eric. *Fast Food Nation*. New York: Harper Perennial, 2005.

Stubbe, Henry. *The Indian Nectar, or, A Discourse Concerning Chocolata*. London: Andrew Crook, 1662.

Tannahill, Reay. *Food in History*. New York: Three Rivers Press, 1988.

Tuebner, Christian, Leopold Forsthofer, Silvio Rizzi, Sybil Grafin Schonfeldt, Karl Schumacher, and Eckart Witzigmann. *The Chocolate Bible: The Definitive Sourcebook*. New York: Penguin Studio, 1997.

Wybauw, Jean-Pierre. *Fine Chocolate, Great Experiences*. France: Lannoo, 2006.

Yard, Sherry. *The Secrets of Baking*. New York: Houghton Mifflin, 2003.

Young, Allen M. *The Chocolate Tree: A Natural History of Cacao*. Gainsville, FL: University Press of Florida, 2007.

index